OUT THE BACK WITH
BONDI RESCUE

True stories behind the hit TV show

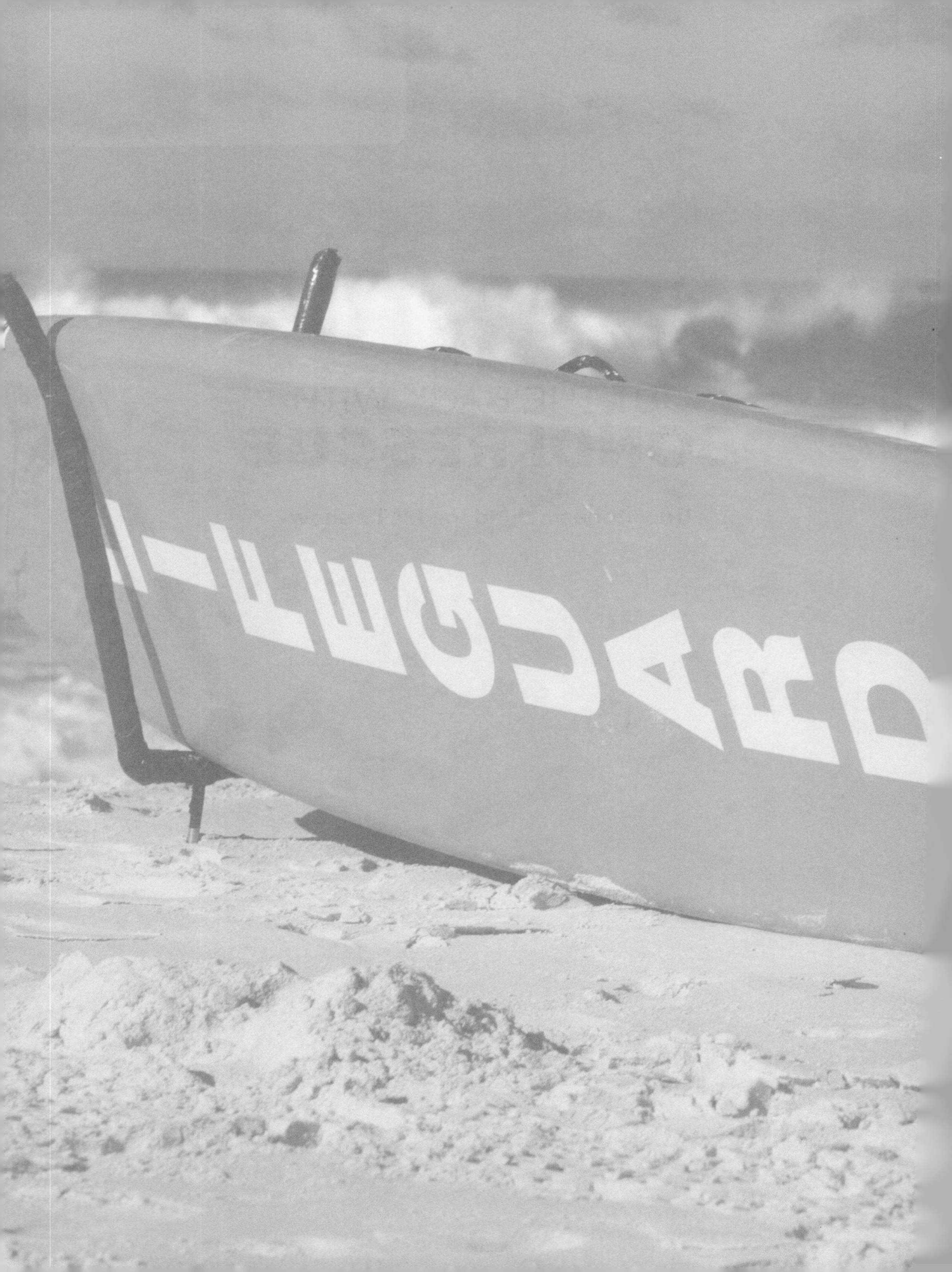

OUT THE BACK WITH

BONDI RESCUE

True stories behind the hit TV show

Nick Carroll

Principal photographer: Bill Morris

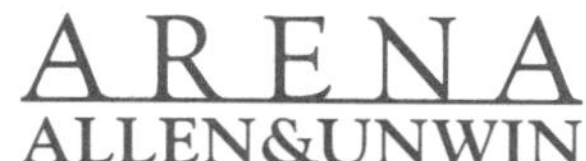

First published in 2009

Arena, an imprint of
Allen & Unwin
83 Alexander Street
Crows Nest NSW 2065
Australia
Phone: (61 2) 8425 0100
Fax: (61 2) 9906 2218
Email: info@allenandunwin.com
Web: www.allenandunwin.com

Cataloguing-in-Publication details are available from
the National Library of Australia
www.librariesaustralia.nla.gov.au

ISBN 978 1 74175 908 2

Internal design by Avril Makula, Gravity AAD
Printed in Australia by McPherson's Printing Group

Photographs
Commissioned photographs are copyright © Bill Morris
Other photographs are courtesy of the lifeguards and their families
and are reproduced with permission

10 9 8 7 6 5 4 3 2 1

Produced under Licence from Cordell Jigsaw Productions

Cordell jigsaw

CONTENTS

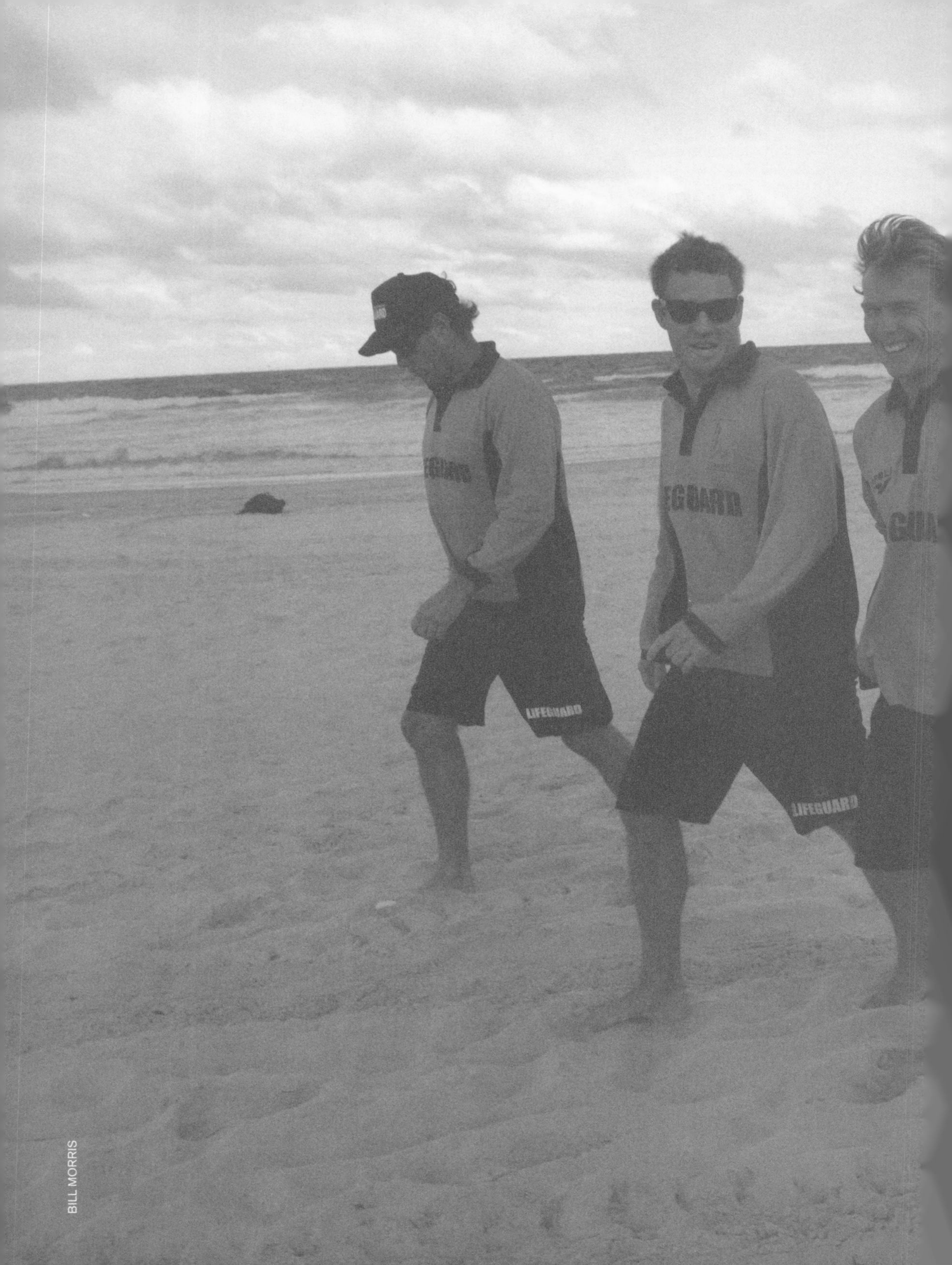

BILL MORRIS

1
ACCIDENTAL STARS

In the land of sandcastles, they're the kings

Here's the paradox at the heart of these blokes' existence: not one of 'em set out to be on TV. Old friends of Rod Kerr's (better known as 'Kerrbox', or just plain 'Box') still can't believe he's appearing in publicity shoots and being invited to glossy Sydney social occasions. Anthony 'Harries' Carroll can't believe his luck. Corey Oliver finds it most amusing. Reidy's busy taking photos, or running the ATV (All-terrain Vehicle). Tommy 'Egg' Bunting is in a Bachelor of the Year contest and isn't even sure why. Deano Gladstone tries his best to shrug the whole thing off, Ryan 'Whippet' Clark has already been there, and Bruce 'Hoppo' Hopkins juggles the roster pretty much as if *Bondi Rescue* had never gone to air.

Yet here they are, almost out of nowhere, accidental stars of a show that puts them on a million and a half Australian TV screens and wins Logie Awards in the process.

There's plenty of reality-based documentary television being made, but none seems to strike quite the same sunny chord as *Bondi Rescue* and its squad of laconic water-boys. How'd this happen? How'd they get here, and what difference has it made to their lives? This book gives us a chance to find out more about the key members of Bondi's lifeguard echelon, and what it takes to become part of what they call 'the service'.

As you'll find out in the pages ahead, there's quite a bit more to both the service and the crew than meets the eye. Today's Bondi lifeguard is at the modern end of a long line of characters, some of them larrikins, some martinets, some wayward, some hard-cases, yet all devoted to something truly, iconically Australian, something we've shaped in our own image now for a century—the beach and surf culture.

They'd be doing this work whether the TV cameras were on or not, and it'd be no less important either way.

They look after a piece of coast that's seen generations of us swim, surf, half-drown, be attacked by bluebottles and sharks, make fools and heroes of ourselves, and most of all, have an incredible load of classic Australian fun.

Maybe this is the show's real charm: their world is our natural playground. In the land of sandcastles, they're the kings.

Then there's the hard underlying fact, the other side of the charm: in this playground they're not always playing games. In an average season, the Bondi lifeguard crew will retrieve several bodies, perform critical resuscitations—which may or may not work—on several more, and keep thousands more people out of possibly serious trouble in the first place. They'd be doing this work whether

RIGHT They're getting used to the camera.
From top: Box, Corey, Reidy, Hoppo, Dean, Harries.

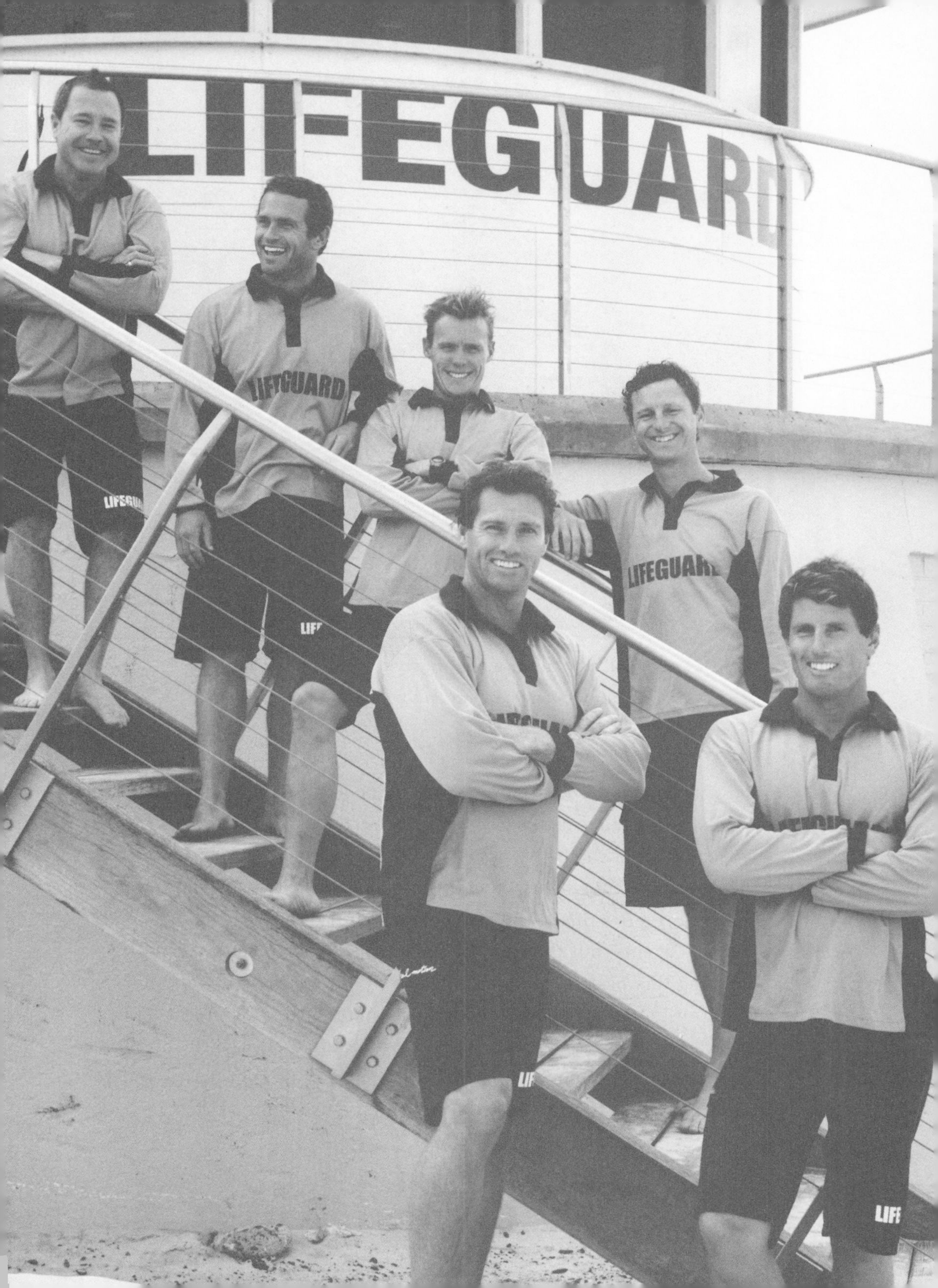

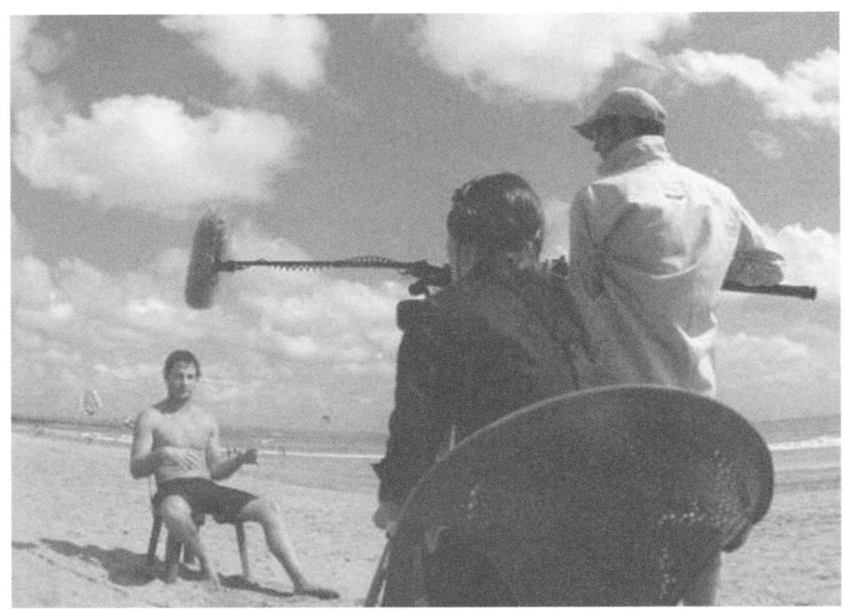

ABOVE It's not always easy relaxing in front of a director and a boom mic; being on the beach helps a lot.

the TV cameras were on or not, and it'd be no less important either way. Reading the many stories within these pages, we're pretty sure, will convince anybody that occasionally these guys do get to be heroes, the actual real thing, and when they do, it sure isn't an accident.

And there's the setting. The world's full of airports, cops and customs agents, but there's only one Bondi Beach. The last day of shooting this past season was a Thursday in late March, well after the frantic 40,000-strong crowds of January. A thunderstorm had just passed inland over the city and the rain had cleared the air; a gorgeous rich late light from the falling sun cast itself across the buildings and cliffs. Bondi, the half-infamous haunt of rich men

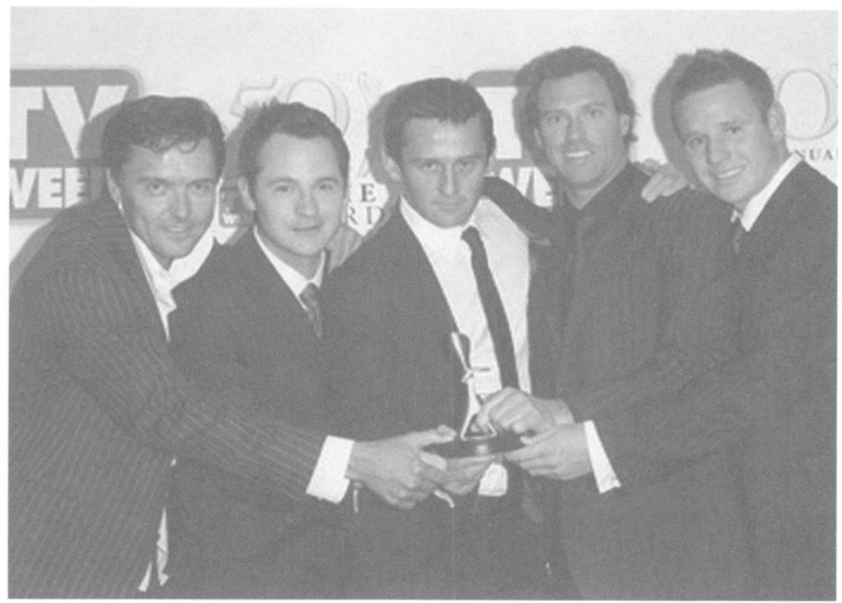

ABOVE Second time's the charm. Show creator Ben Davies (centre) with some of his characters, Logie Awards 2009.

and rogues, was glowing, only a couple of hundred people wandering its sands. Tom Bunting, seated in one of the ATVs near the flags, relaxed—well, as much as any lifeguard relaxes. Nobody was going under this arvo; it was just too beautiful. 'You can't buy this,' he said, and he's right.

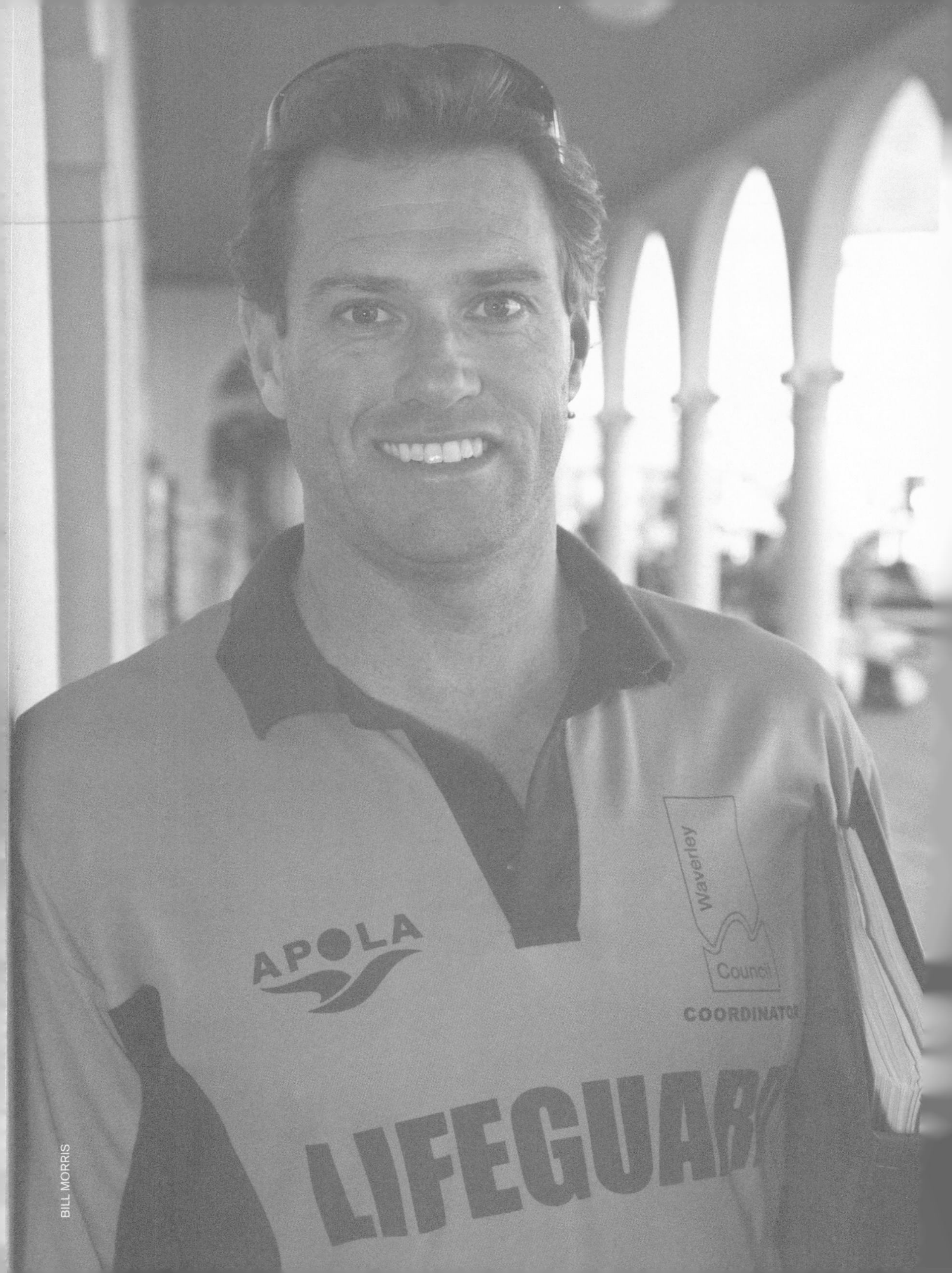

BILL MORRIS

Hoppo: The Boss
(Bruce Hopkins)

'They're starting to nickname me "The Florist",' Bruce Hopkins says, starting to grin, 'cos I'm making my own arrangements.'

Hoppo's sitting at a coffee-shop table just behind the Bondi Pavilion, and pondering the mechanisms by which he—a quiet kid, unsure of the water—has come to feature in the Sydney papers' society columns and make speeches at Logie Awards nights.

In a sense Hoppo—40 years of age, fit, sharp and serious—is where the modern Bondi lifeguard begins and ends. He came to the job when it was teetering between its past larrikinism and its future as an actual profession, when it needed someone willing to mould it into what Hoppo and his fellow lifeguards can now unblushingly call a 'service'.

And he was the right man for the task, partly because he's that very simple thing—a local. Underneath the façade of this busy, urban, tourist-driven area, communities are ticking away, as they have been for a century, and that's where Hoppo and the boys on his team have come from—not out of the Sunday social pages or the TV guides, but out of the eastern suburbs bedrock.

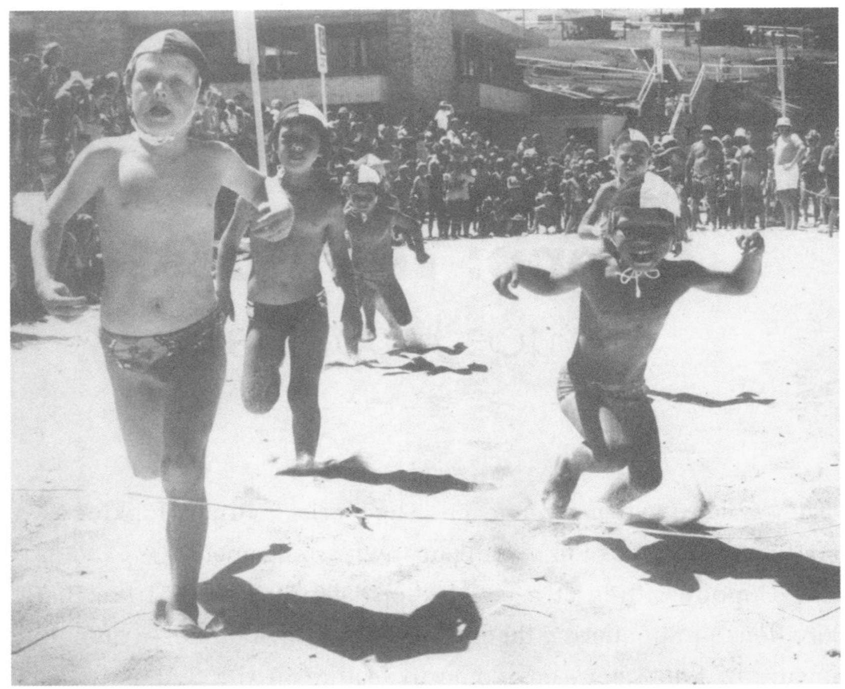

ABOVE Kind of a competitive Nipper. Six-year-old Hoppo plunges for the line at Bronte Beach.

Bruce might well have been a country boy instead. His father, Aden, now retired, grew up in Crookwell, just north of Goulburn, and moved to Sydney as a teenager. He was a baker by trade who worked for a couple of decades as a golf-club maker for Slazenger and another couple of decades as a Brambles security bloke. He was also a passionate sportsman who played field hockey for many years, barely missed Olympic selection, and eventually needed a hip replacement at the age of 60. Mum Joan was born in Coffs Harbour, and came to Sydney when her foreman father was transferred.

hoppo the boss

Bruce Aden Hopkins came into the world at Paddington Women's Hospital on 12 November 1968. A few years later he was joined by younger brother Mark. Joan and Aden had a place in Leichhardt Street, Charing Cross, next to St Catherine's School, between Bondi and Bronte. Joan, a housewife at first, became interested in swim coaching after putting the kids through backyard swim school, started coaching in the St Catherine's pool, and made a 30-year career out of it.

By way of contrast, Bruce's dad was 'self-taught in the river'. Hoppo says, 'They just threw each other in. You had to teach yourself right then, or go under.'

Aden had joined South Maroubra surf club for a while, but the kids went to Bronte when the parents realised they needed to be educated about surf. Thus, Hoppo joined Bronte Nippers at the age of six, and, in what might be seen as one of those horrific life-defining events, met Rod Kerr. Rodney was in the under-7s, and according to Hoppo, 'Nothing's changed!'

Hoppo was afraid of the ocean at first. 'Dad was a real hard-arse Aussie country type of bloke, you know, "Just get in and do it, what's this about fear? Out you go!" Dad would jump in and do water safety with Box's old man; there were some pretty good watermen around us. But I remember sometimes I really didn't wanna go in. I'd be paddling out on these little nipper boards and my head'd be higher than a kite, craning off the board looking at what was coming next … I think anyone who saw me at eleven years old and was told what I'd end up doing, they'd have said, "No way".'

He ran in the club's beach sprint and relay races, played hockey, was good at cricket, but the water didn't leak into his head until later in his teens. At the time there was a bit of a divide between the surf club and hardcore surfers. The surfers would hang out at The Den, just across the other side of the beach, smoking dope, drinking; then there were the surf-club kids, some of them would surf a bit, and they'd hang out at the clubhouse. Bruce would sit there while Kerrbox and his mates charged out, caught a million waves, and came in bagging each other. Over time, one way or another, he realised he'd have to go out there too.

Hoppo, with his blue eyes and square jaw, can come across as a near-cliché of the Aussie male ... But there's more to him than that.

Hoppo went to rough-and-tumble Dover Heights High, filling up as it was at the time with lots of big New Zealanders who'd just come across the Tasman. On his first day at the school, he and a mate caught the bus that passed near Hoppo's place, and there was no-one on the bus. 'We thought, "Beauty, let's sit down the back." Not knowing that at the next bus stop there'd be a crew of Year 11 and 12 kids waiting, and down the back was their hang. We got kicked up the arse the whole way down.

'That year, I got bashed every time I got on the bus. I'd come home with bruises on my shins and arms and Mum would go "What's this?" and I'd say "Nah, nothing". Couldn't say too much cos she'd be running up to school and then I'd get it worse!' He laughs, but knows it was a tough time.

Hoppo did 'enough to get by' at school, and had a great work-experience week with an uncle, Bill Jenkings, who was a crime reporter on the notorious old Sydney *Daily Mirror*. It whetted his appetite for media and Hoppo ended up carrying the microphone at games for the Greg Hartley/Peter Peters League show on 2GB, which he loved. Another option in his mind was the water police, but that never came close to eventuating.

Well past his resistance to water, he got into surf-ski paddling and ironman racing, with considerable success. Hoppo, with his clear blue eyes, square jaw, and general sense of practical, healthy manhood, can come across as a near-clichéd image of the Aussie male lifeguard. But there is more to Hoppo than there seems at first glance. He watches people quite closely through those clear eyes, doesn't blink, chooses his words. He's watched the lifeguard service in Waverley change massively since he was hired as a casual nearly 20 years ago. 'When I first started I thought I'll do five years and then move on once I got the Senior Lifeguard title. But now … I'm still here!

'In those days, a lot of the time you'd work on your own. My first day, at Tamarama, I got handed a pair of shorts, a shirt, a whistle, and a couple of badges that I had to sew on myself. And I'm down there at Tama first day on my own … There'd be times when you'd be finishing on your own in an arvo with 15,000 people on the beach. At least you're your own boss.' At the time there might have been ten or twelve guards compared to today's 36.

Back then lifeguarding wasn't treated as a profession: 'You were a beach bum, or it was something you did in between doing something else, before you got a real job.' Yet it had its own problems. There was a lot more council ordinance work, a kind of policing job chasing down minor by-law offences: dogs on the beach, incidents on the promenade, skateboarders, that sort of thing. The sort of jobs the council rangers do these days. There were crowds coming down to the beach, but not so many constantly in the water putting themselves in endless need of rescue. And, Hoppo says, 'There were nowhere near the same numbers of surf schools as today.'

Hoppo doesn't recall the 1994 Boxing Day riots, when the park and the Esplanade were swamped by lunatic drunks, but he does recall the 1994 bushfires, when Sydney was literally ringed by flames. 'You could see waves breaking, then see the ash surface in the foam. The sun went down in this amazing orange glow, but it was dark because of the smoke. Ash was everywhere. There was a really eerie feeling about it.'

And he remembers the solo rescues. Like the time he went out on a board in heavy surf to grab an Englishman in trouble, got him on the board, then was pitch-poled by an 8-foot wave into shallow sand. 'In those days the old blokes used to say, "Never let go of the rescue board!" I hung on and the board went straight into the sand and the force went directly through my shoulders.' Hoppo felt his left shoulder dislocate. He came up and the Englishman surfaced right next to him. 'I told him "Hang on", and I sorta shuffled the board halfway round to shore—we were facing out to sea. Another wave was coming and I had to sit back and push. When it hit, the jerk of it pushed the shoulder back in! I've come in and the Pommy bloke got up, didn't say thanks or anything, and I've got three months in a sling trying to get the shoulder right.

'But it's a fine line. We're lucky, I s'pose. Most of the time it's been big, I've been able to come through it OK.'

The beach-bum era flowed along for a while into the 1980s and early 1990s. Aside from the council ordinance work, the lifeguards were pretty much left to run the place how they liked; that was the way it'd always been done, and as a result, Hoppo explains, it became a private kingdom on the beach. Nobody oversaw the overtime logs or the expenditures. There was no formalised testing for the job beyond an 800-metre timed swim; no M-shape course, no rescue

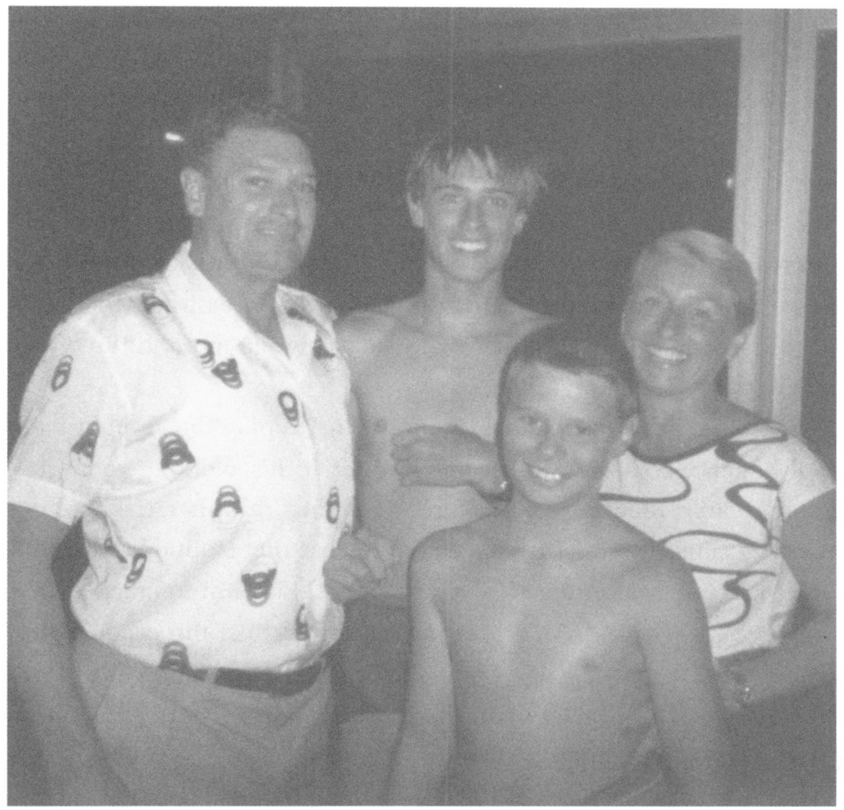

ABOVE Nothing like the beach to keep teenage boys occupied. The Hopkinses: Aden, Bruce, Mark and Joan.

skills updates. Naturally enough, compared with today's tight ship, lifeguard discipline was pretty wobbly.

'There's no way they could've done the show back then,' says Hoppo, cringing at the idea. 'It would all have come out … it'd have been an embarrassment.'

In 2000, the Surf Life Saving Association (SLSA) started trying to set up its own professional lifeguard service, and began bidding for Waverley's business. Hoppo, along with fellow guard Lawrie Williams, was called in by the council guy who told him, 'You've got eight months to fix this up, or I'm signing their contract.'

Hoppo took the head job, and with Williams's help, time and effort saw the lifeguard culture change. Tests and skills were certified, and a new crop of younger, surf-tuned guards were hired. Gradually, as things developed, the lifeguards' focus swung more to the water, where today it's firmly fixed.

The process has meant Hoppo having to play the straight man, the leader who keeps his team on course. It's worked; today the guards carry themselves like pros. Yet they're still larrikins, and there's a sense in how they speak of the boss that Hoppo battles a bit of a larrikin streak himself. They're waiting for him to crack. 'I saw him have a few drinks the other night,' Harries will chortle, and they'll all join in, like schoolboys joking about a favourite teacher.

'The show's given me a bit more life as a lifeguard ... and it's opened more doors outside lifeguarding.'

His team all talk about doing the job forever, but as Hoppo says: 'There's a time limit ... the body begins to break down. You can't do all this training and go surfing and everything and expect it to last. When you're in your twenties, it's the best job in the world. You come down to the beach, hang out, talk with your mates, watch the surf. Once you get into your forties, and you've got a couple of kids, you start wondering.'

Interestingly, Bruce Hopkins is in that exact position; he's nursing a torn hamstring after trying to run hard in a sand sprint, and he's getting more involved in other areas—media, the lifeguards' clothing offshoot, managing the guards' involvement with the show. His own arrangements, as 'The Florist' puts it. And he has those couple of kids—girls, who decorate his office with pictures of Dad on TV.

Where does it all leave him now? 'The show's given me a bit more life as a lifeguard,' he says seriously. 'And it's opened more doors outside lifeguarding, dealing more in the business world. But I still need lifeguarding to make that work. It's all connected.'

wild stories FROM THE SERVICE

Self-preservation

WHEN DOES A lifeguard preserve himself above the rescue? Bruce Hopkins has an answer to that one. He's considered letting go only once, on a big-surf day at Bronte, when he and a barely conscious patient were drifting outside the rocks. On big days at those beaches, you don't even bother trying to get back to the beach you came from, you just let yourself get swept to the next beach—Tamarama to Bronte in a north swell, vice versa in a south. 'I had this bloke, I got hold of him with the tube,' describes Hoppo, 'and we were just getting thumped.' They were caught in a kind of nightmare familiar to surfers in big waves—a washing-machine cycle on the rim of a shallow sandbank, where one wave would hit and push them in, the next would suck them back out to the sandbank rim again, pound, suck, pound, suck, with no way out until the ocean decided to ease off. Hoppo says, 'He was doing nothing, he was conscious but making no effort—the rescue tube was all that was keeping him up. I had flippers on but I was having to grab him after every wave and haul him back up, and I was getting tired. Holding my breath, diving under foam, hauling him up again. I thought, "If this doesn't let up soon, I'm gonna have to let him go and get myself out of it".' Hoppo decided through his fatigue to hang in for another minute or so, then the waves let up, and he was able to get them both clear and out of danger. Back on the beach he found the man's eight-year-old son, panicking. He is still haunted by the idea of what he'd have said to the kid if he'd cut loose his dad.

I nearly destroyed Richard Branson

SIR RICHARD BRANSON, the well-known British entrepreneur, is a frequent visitor to Bondi and an exceptionally canny exploiter of both the scenery and the press. One day his people somehow inveigle Hoppo into taking Sir Richard for a jet-ski ride. 'He was on the sled, and the photographer asked me to drive in close to the beach and whip it around, so he could take a shot of Branson with spray everywhere and this big expression on his face. So I did it, but I did it too hard,' Hoppo confesses. 'I did it so hard the ski spun around and kept going, and so did the sled. We both went over the side ... we were lucky the water wasn't any shallower, or we'd have been really damaged.' Ah well, he's supposed to be a thrillseeker.

Sir Galahad of Bondi

HUMAN NATURE ISN'T always seen at its finest during a surf rescue at Bondi. It's midsummer and Hoppo spots a couple—husband and wife—in trouble. He jumps in to get them, thinking it isn't anything out of the ordinary ... but it is. 'When I got to them, the husband had his hands clamped on her shoulders and he was trying to keep himself afloat by holding her underwater. She was down there underneath just holding her breath. You could tell in his eyes he didn't have any idea what he was doing, he was in panic mode and doing whatever he could to stop from going under too.' Hoppo snaps the husband into focus, loads them on and takes them back to the beach. 'I dunno if they're still married,' he says dryly. 'She was FURIOUS with him. Back on the sand she was tearing into him ... he was just saying, "Honest, I didn't know what was happening!"'

How Hoppo lost his surf ski

A GOOD RACING surf ski is worth a fair slab of cash—anywhere between two and three grand, depending on who your friends are. Hoppo has good friends, so his skis come in around the two-grand mark. A few winters ago, a large humpback whale on an early migration path decided to take a few weeks off; it swam into the harbour, spent a week there, then came back around the corner and wallowed away two weeks just cruising around inside Bondi Bay. If it'd been summer, the whale would've been mobbed, but as it was, her fan club restrained itself to beach views and the odd accidental approach via a bay swim. That is until Hoppo and a mate decided to take their skis and have a stickybeak from the surface angle. 'We paddled out OK, she was out off the north end, then as we approached she just went under,' he says. 'We were thinking, "Hey, where's she gone?" Then she comes up right between us!' The whale must have decided to take a look at them instead. Suddenly realising they were at risk of a wallop from the whale's flukes, Hoppo and his mate quickly headed south, but as they did so, a big set of waves reared up. Hoppo recalls, 'By now we were in front of Icebergs ... the waves were getting bigger and finally one reared up bigger than all the rest and I just scraped over it, but he didn't. I started laughing until I turned around and there was the biggest of the lot.' Hoppo lost his ski and it rolled straight onto the rocks and snapped perfectly in two. 'I can't believe whale-watching cost me two grand.'

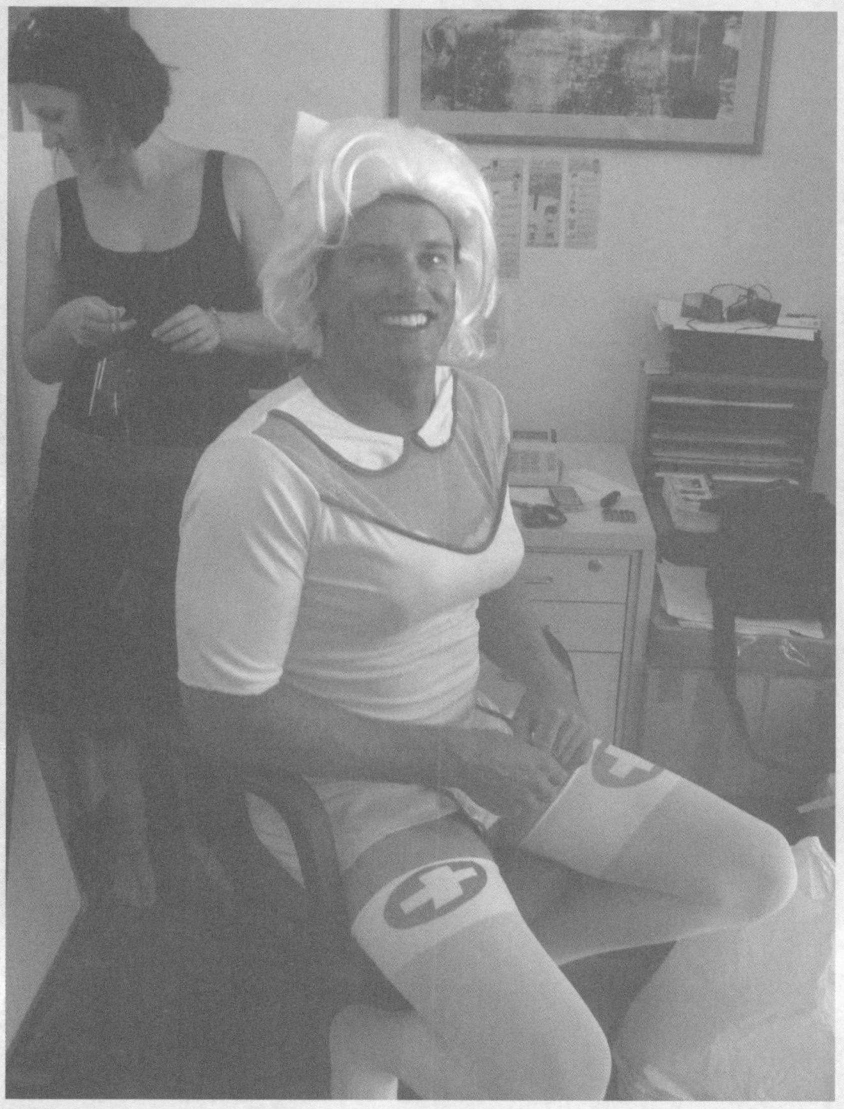

ABOVE When it comes to community contributions, for the Bondi boys, there's just no limit. Hoppo doing his best nurse imitation for a local fundraiser.

2
THE JOB

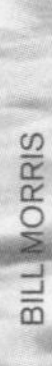

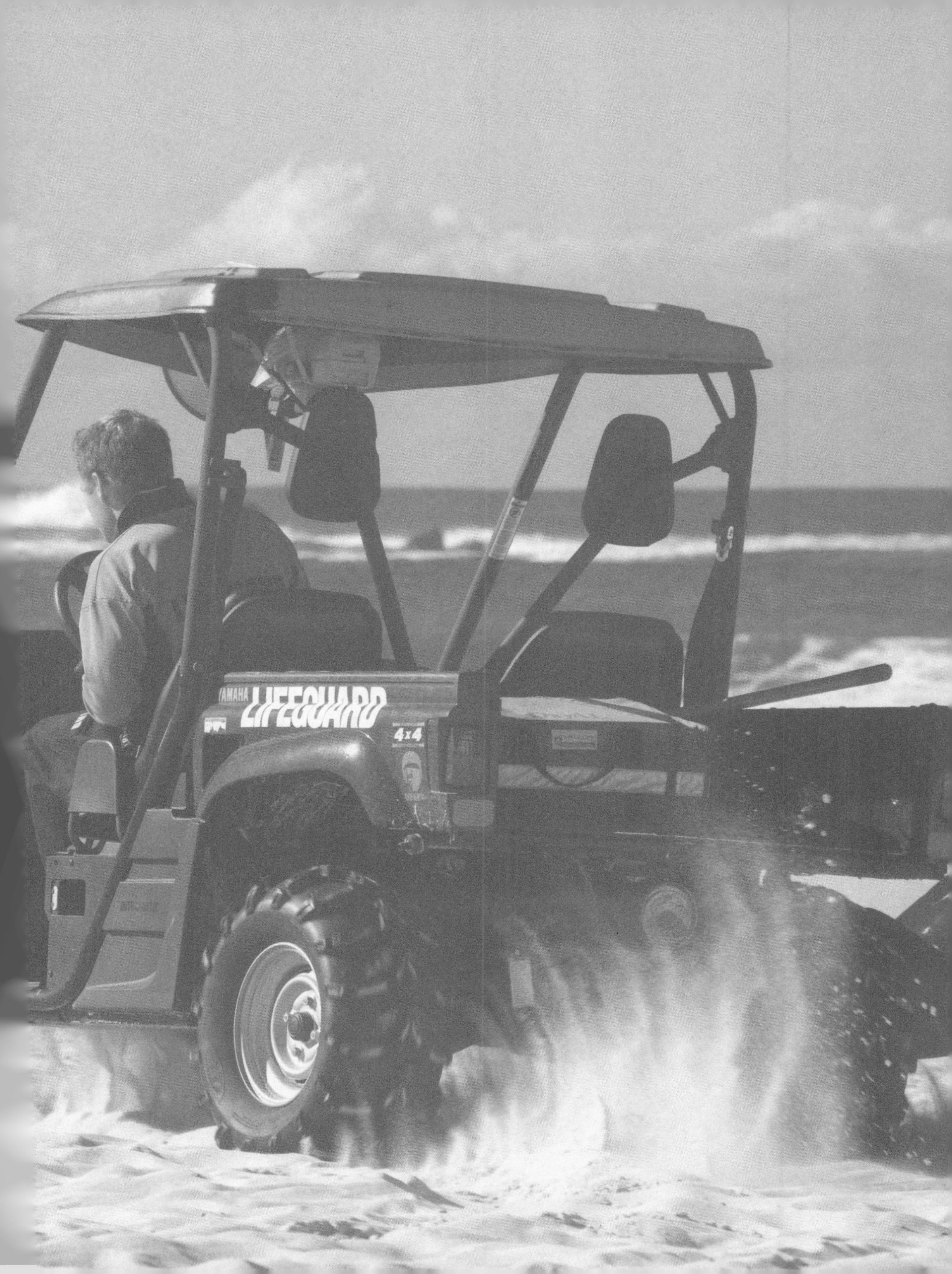
YAMAHA
LIFEGUARD
4x4

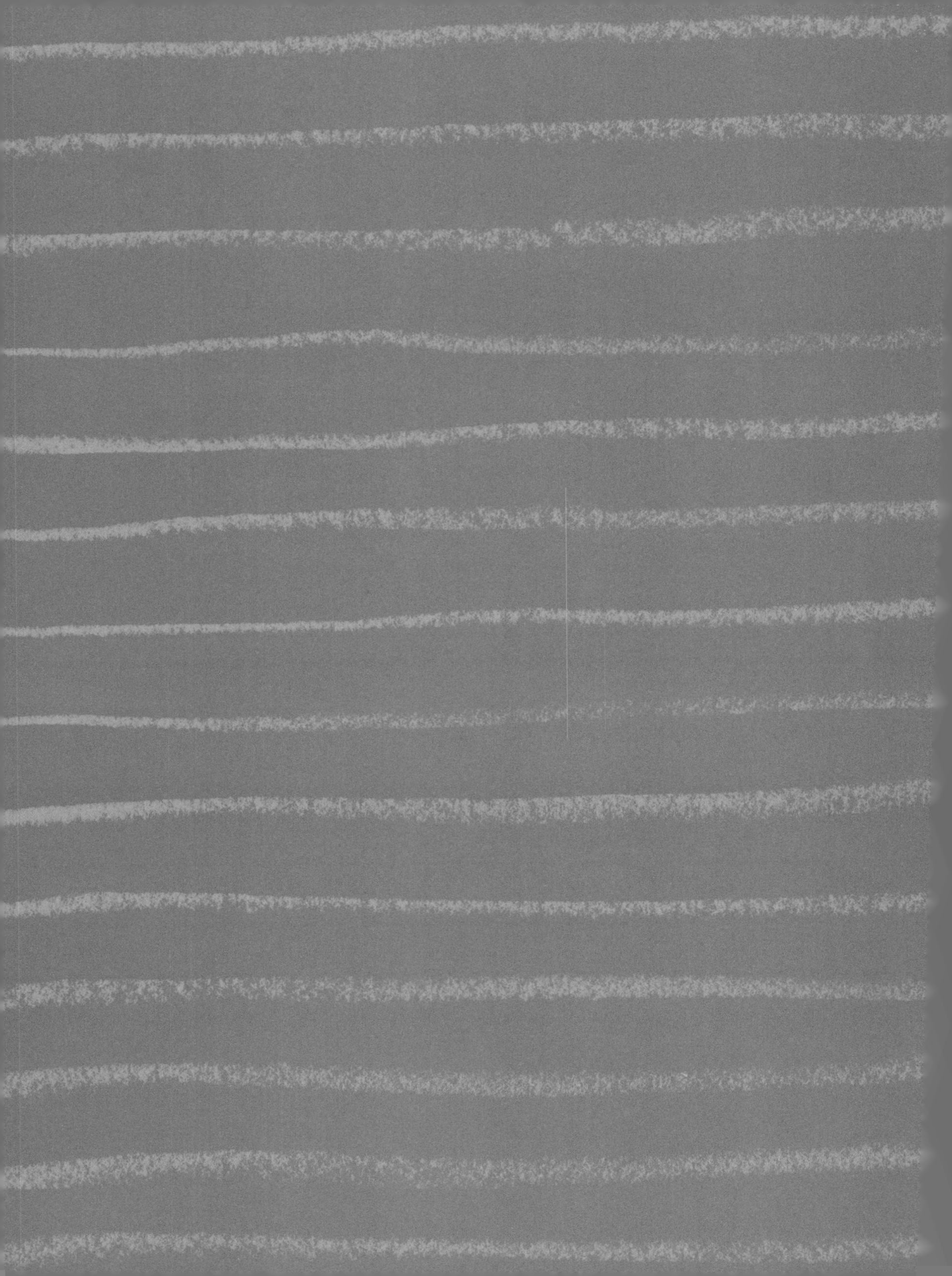

What it is, what it was, and how it's changed

Twenty-one dollars an hour. An extra four dollars once you've worked your way up. If you're a prospective lifeguard candidate for Waverley Council, that should pour a little chilly seawater on your dreams of wealth and fame.

Still, it's not bad compared with the five pounds a week earned in 1913 by Dennis 'Dinny' Brown, Bondi's first professional lifeguard.

'Five pounds,' muses veteran lifeguard Lawrie Williams. 'Actually, that might not have sounded too bad back then.'

Lawrie is the Bondi lifeguard service's unofficial keeper of the flame. On the beach himself since 1978, he's spent a considerable part of his spare time in the past couple of years digging up facts on the likes of Dinny Brown. The small, fascinating strand of Australian history now in Lawrie's charge goes part-way to explaining how one bloke and five pounds a week eventually became a 36-person service, and a top-rated Australian TV series.

Professional lifeguarding in Australia began at Manly in 1903. Prior to that, the beaches were combed by 'nuisance inspectors', whose punitive tasks included booting out those reckless citizens who dared to swim after 7 a.m. When swimmers were first allowed to bathe during daylight hours and the council realised it needed to

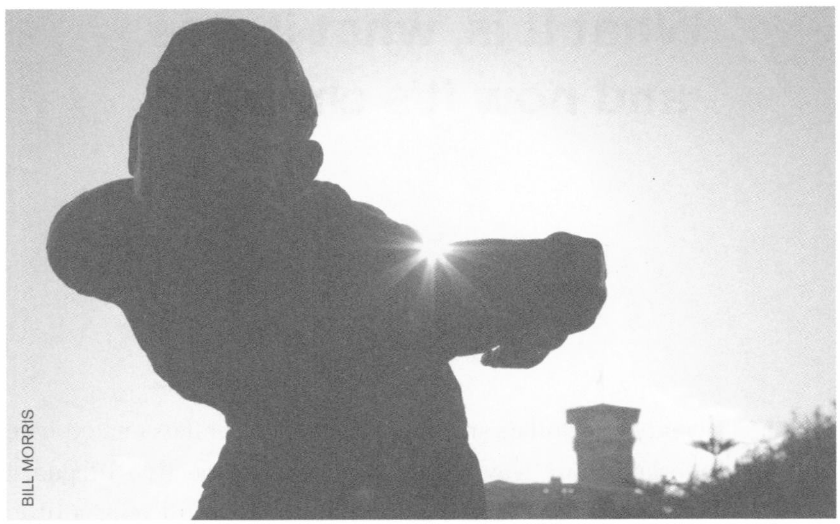

ABOVE Part of the heritage. The famous Bondi lifesaver statue just south of the pavilion.

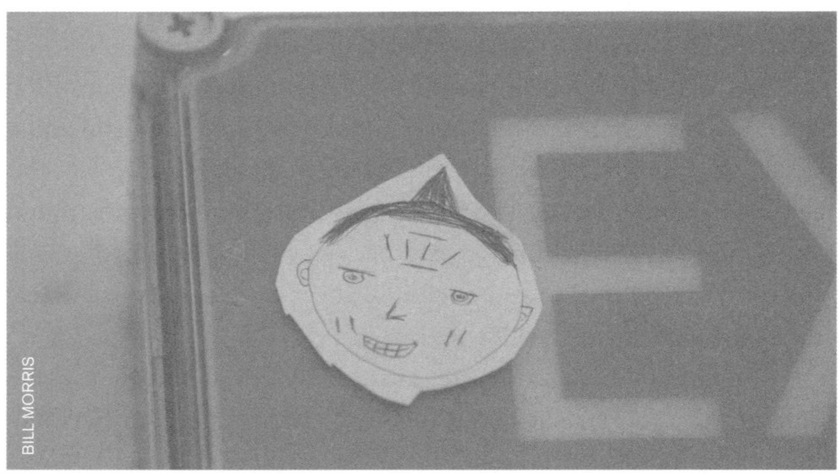

ABOVE Part of the endless piss-take. Whippet's artistic impression of Box's amazing head.

supply some sort of protection, they hired the Sly brothers, members of a famous aquatically oriented local family, who had the good fortune to own a large rowing boat. The Slys' efforts preceded Manly's first volunteer patrol club by three years.

At Bondi, the volunteer club preceded the pros by seven summers. As a result, when Waverley Council decided to employ a 'full-time lifesaver' to cover the non-volunteer hours, they turned to the Bondi Surf Bathers Life Saving Club (SBLSC) for recommendations. And there was Dinny, a Bronte local who joined the surf club probably in order to get the job. His father was a Waverley alderman, which may also have helped.

Dennis lasted at Bondi until 1923, at which time he took over the Bronte surf sheds and their hiring concessions. His son Dave, a legendary Eastern Suburbs rugby league player, took over the sheds when Dennis retired, and ran them till the 1960s. And the Bondi SBLSC's recommendation remained the lifeguards' selection process all the way to the 1990s.

At Bondi, Dennis was joined by Stan McDonald, who stayed until 1933. Stan was a big New Zealander who had a near-cult following—he once won the title of 'Most Popular Man in Bondi', no doubt a hard-fought contest. Like Dennis, Stan went on to run a beach concession—the blow-up mats, the icy-poles, the spray-on mutton-bird oil tanning lotion.

There were no rescue boards or tubes back then. To effect a rescue, the guards used a reel, line and belt. If in need, they'd recruit people off the beach to assist. If they were working 'one-out', they'd go out by themselves.

Sharks were more prevalent in those days; they appear in many of the bravery awards issued to Waverley lifeguards by the Royal Humane Society. 'The tiger sharks used to swim all the way down the cliffs at the north end, then the guys down there would catch 'em off the boat ramp,' says Bruce Hopkins. He tells a story—perhaps a Bondi myth—about a lifeguard in the 1920s who, having spotted someone in trouble off the north end, hurled on the belt and went charging out with a line trailing. On the way out, the lifeguard swam right past a big shark which was being hauled the other way by a fisherman.

The guards remained 'full-time lifesavers' until the 1940s, when the role began to include council by-law enforcement. Then they became known as 'beach inspectors'—shades of that old nuisance-inspector title. Aub Laidlaw, the most famous of all the Bondi beach inspectors, was born in 1909, was on the beach by 1929, and quit in 1969—an unfathomable stretch of time, spanning a huge shift in demographics, wealth, behaviour and public morality. For many years he was a hero, but by the end of his time, says Lawrie, Aub was an anachronism: 'Everything had changed around him, and he hadn't changed a bit ... it must have been difficult.' Aub was followed by Allen Johnston, whose sturdy conservative approach made him a target of active harassment from skateboarding kids and the surfing 'Bush Hill Gang'.

When surfer Brad Mayes (son of Bondi surf legend Jack 'Bluey' Mayes) was appointed a lifeguard in the late 1970s, it signalled the first move away from Bondi SBLSC's strict control over the job. By the mid-1990s, when Kerrbox was signed up, the shift was well underway. Simply: surfers were fantastic at reading the water, they could see things coming a mile away. As Lawrie Williams, a long-time surfer himself, says, 'They were great in the water—as long as they got to work on time.'

The 'beach inspector' name lasted until 1994, when it was officially changed to 'lifeguard'.

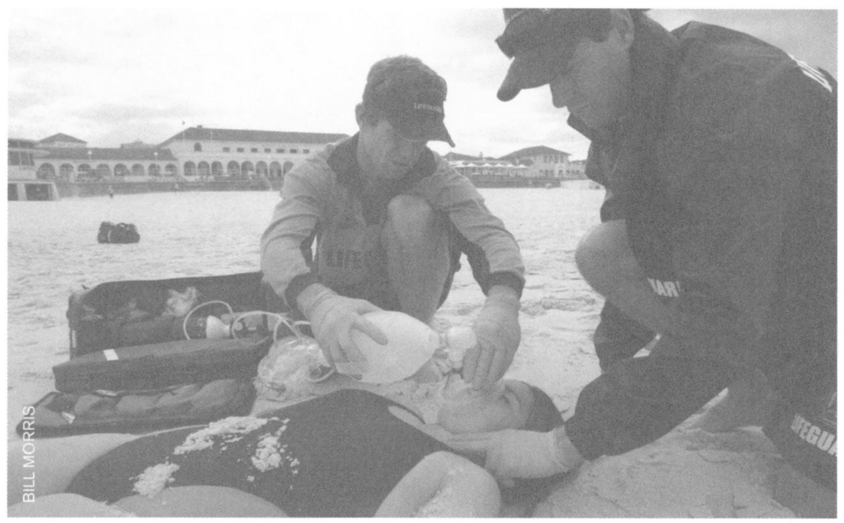

ABOVE This is what they mean by 'bagging'– the Oxy-viva therapy system in full swing.

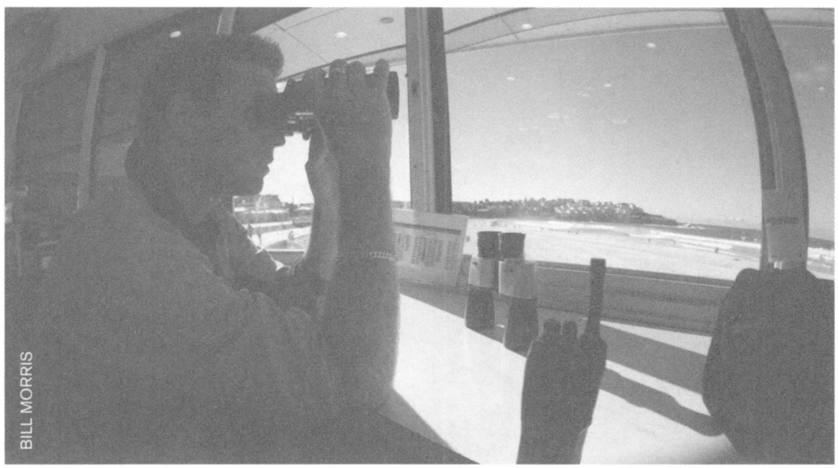

ABOVE Someone's always got to be in the tower. Whippet, eyes peeled for trouble.

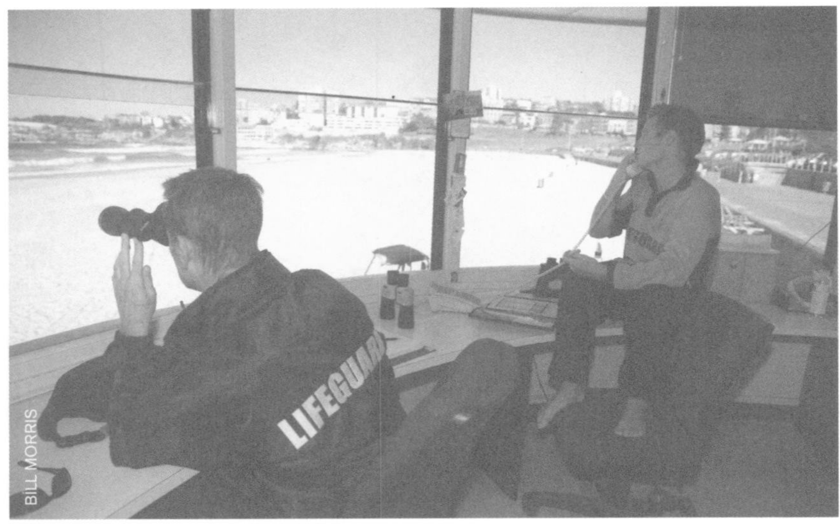

ABOVE The tower is the lifeguards' retreat–lunchroom, hangout and op centre all in one.

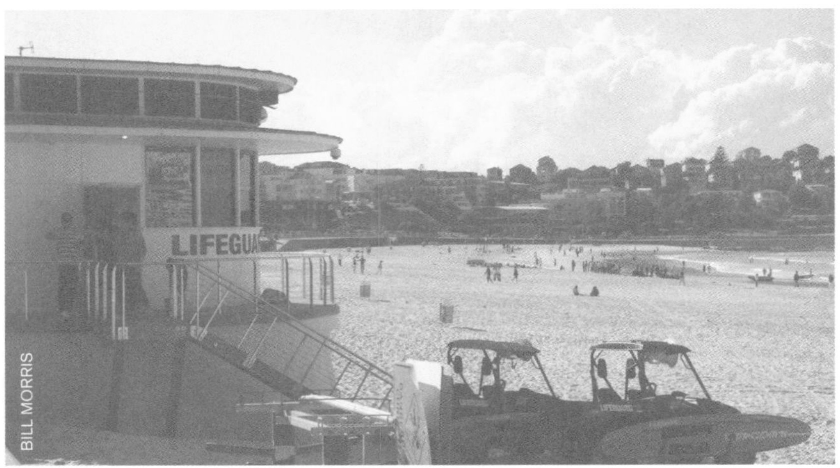

ABOVE In the past decade, council's upped the gear support. 'Rhino' ATVs at the ready.

These days, the world is rich with public liability issues. Not long ago the council lost a case brought against them by a quadriplegic diving victim. Now they have to go to London to get public liability cover for the beach. It's a big part of what's caused the Bondi lifeguards to raise their skill levels and professionalism to modern levels. Bondi's high watermark crowd today is around 60,000—a number that's been more or less steady since the late 1920s. (In Dennis Brown's day, it might've peaked around 10,000.) But the crowd, with the times, has changed. There's a huge range of nationalities, water-skill levels and cultural spreads. With the improvement in the service, people have become more reliant on the lifeguards. This is part of the synergy of *Bondi Rescue*—it's trained people to pay heed to the men in blue.

Hoppo says it's no more crowded now than it was 20 years ago, but that the influx of tourists with their lack of swimming knowledge is what makes today's job a bigger deal. Extra lifeguards started being hired when it became obvious that you couldn't work on your own without incurring serious problems; one lifeguard was nearly drowned after being struck by his own board during a rescue, and was saved by surfers. Over time the council supplied more and more gear. Now Bondi has three ATVs, two jet skis, spinal gear, defibrillators, and a complement of six lifeguards on duty at all times.

Among the many difficulties faced by the lifeguards as they try to figure out their job's new parameters is the relationships with surf clubs. The volunteer surf club patrols are theoretically under the control of the lifeguards, since they have the council's duty of care, but it doesn't always pan out that way. The issue flared in the Sydney press in January 2009, after Box vented frustration on the show at a shark alarm sounded by a club patrol without letting the lifeguards know first. 'That's been one of the most political things,' explains

Hoppo. 'We work in with them and most people in the surf clubs are pretty good. It's more the hierarchy, they have an us-and-them thing and try to portray lifeguards as being anti-surf club, which I dunno why that'd be. Most lifeguards are members of surf clubs, or have been. That's an ongoing battle.'

Then there's the skill that's impossible to teach: the ability to see a situation developing early enough to anticipate it.

The schism is by no means clear-cut. Bronte SLSC, for example, gives an honorary membership to all Waverley Council lifeguards, and Kerrbox goes there for a steak and a beer with the family on weekends. It's not like that at Bondi. 'We have a lot of butting-head problems with the surf clubs,' says Rod. 'It's not the clubs actually, the clubs are cool, it's the higher-ups. Most of the people involved are unreal.'

Perhaps it's affected by another way in which pro lifeguards differ from the lifesavers: The 'clubbies' still suffer to some extent from the long enmity set up in the 1960s and 1970s between surfboard riders and lifesavers. But the lifeguard crew, being core surfers themselves, have very good relationships with skilled local surfers—who do as much as anyone to keep the water safe.

On top of that, says Hoppo, 'I think our level of training and fitness is improving all the time. The way I look at it, it's a professional job, just like an ambo or the police, and you've got to have standards to meet.'

And the standards are toughening all the time. To apply for one of the Waverley positions, you'll need several certificates: a Senior

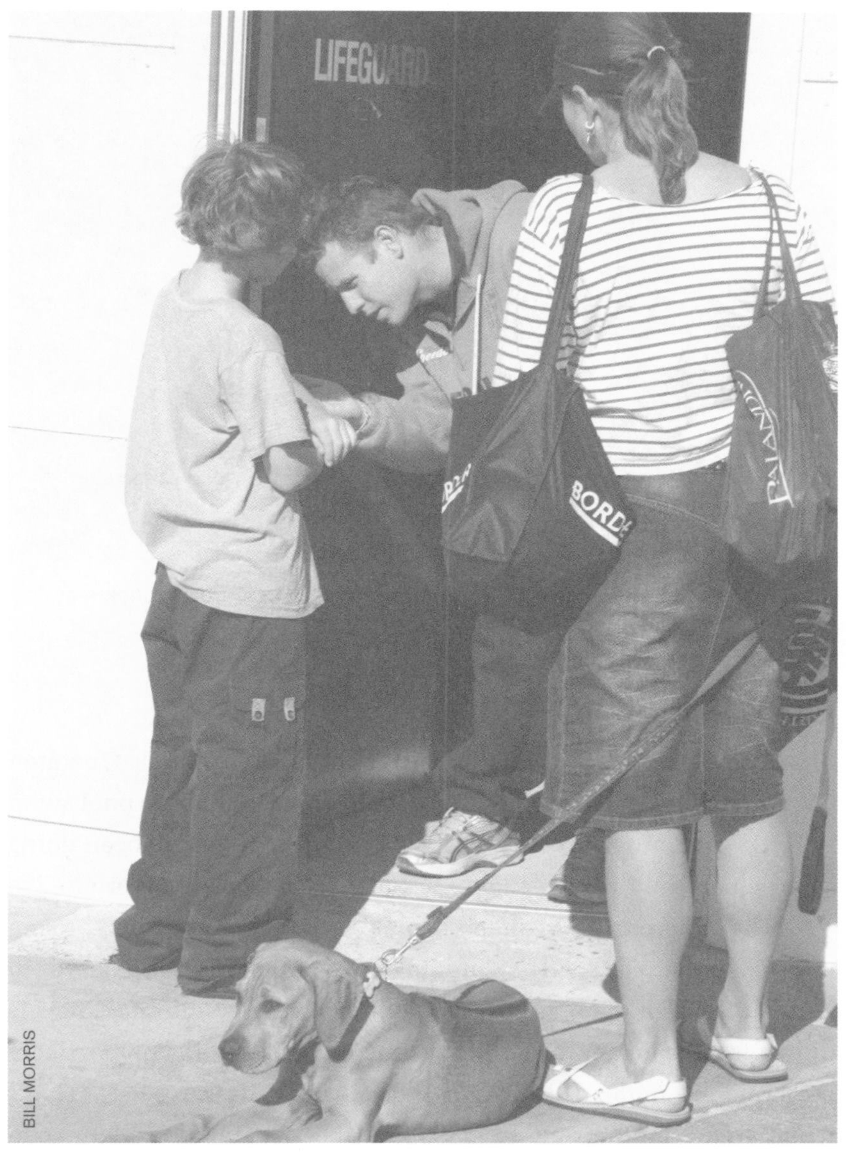

BILL MORRIS

ABOVE You never know who'll need help, or with what. Whippet responds to a skateboarding scratch.

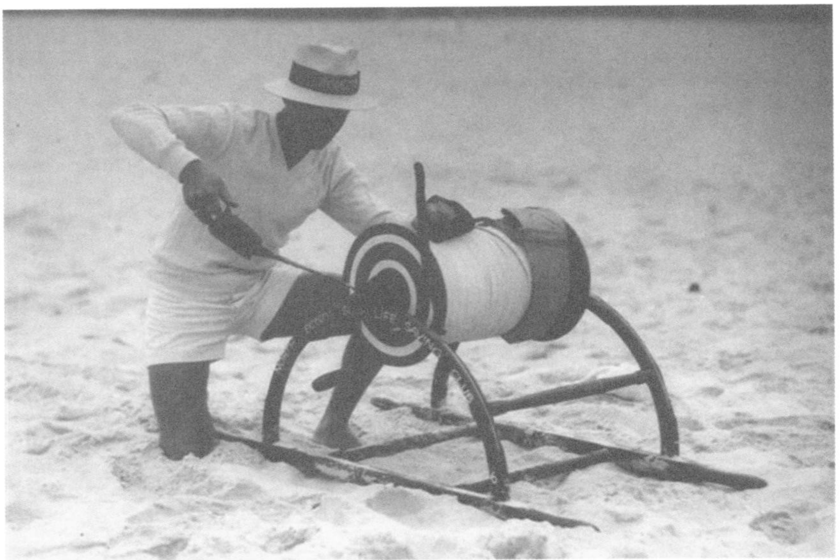

ABOVE The old line-and-belt had one significant drawback–you needed two people to operate it.

First Aid, an Advanced Resuscitation and a Defibrillator Operator. On the water-skills side you'll have to finish an 800-metre pool swim in thirteen minutes. As Reidy says, 'That's fine if you've been doing some squad training, but there's not many who'd do it otherwise.'

Then there's the M-shape course: two 600-metre runs, broken up by 600 metres of surf swimming and 600 metres on a board, in and out through the break all the time, in under 25 minutes. This is drawn from ironman race training, and examines a lifeguard's likely performance under the physical stress of a mass rescue. 'That's when you're more prone to make mistakes, when you're fatigued,' Hoppo says. 'If they can handle that they can handle getting someone in and turning around and doing it again.' To simulate the dead

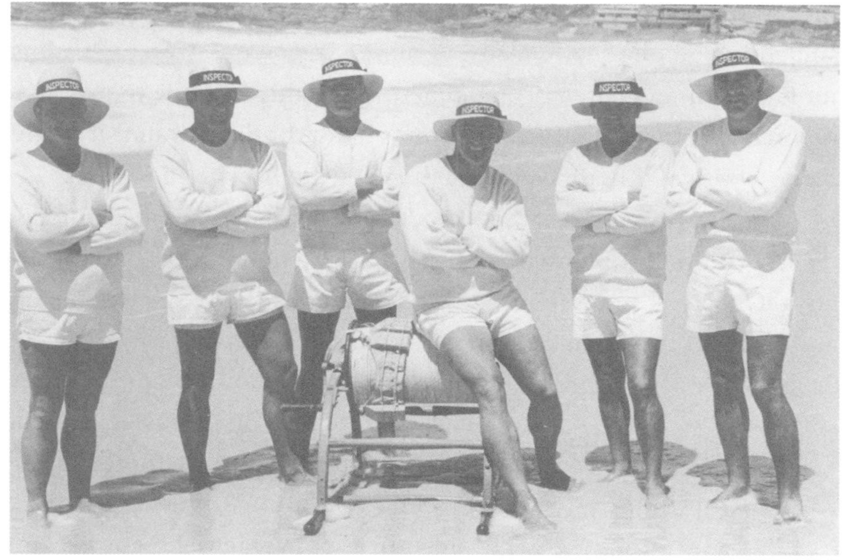

ABOVE Those magnificent men in their gleaming white togs. The Bondi Beach Inspector crew in their 1960s heyday.

weight of an unconscious patient, they use a mannequin weighing about 80 kilos; new recruits have to rescue the mannequin, so they have at least a minor sense of the effort involved.

Then there's a skill Hoppo watches for throughout the testing, something he sees as critical to a good lifeguard, but something he suspects is impossible to teach—the ability to see a situation developing early enough to anticipate it. 'Spotting something that's gonna happen before it happens. That to me is a good lifeguard. It's like a fullback in a footy team. You've got your average fullback and you've got the unreal one. What's the difference? Well, a good one is always in the right position, and when the other team makes a break, there he is. A not-so-good one doesn't see the play developing and the other guys get a try. Same with a good lifeguard. He'll spot something and be there, ready. A more average one won't get going until the thing's already happened. It might be only five or ten seconds but that might be a couple of mouthfuls of water, it might make a critical difference by the time you get back to the beach.'

As Hoppo explains, the tower coordinator's role is also crucial: 'When you're in the tower, you're basically playing chess with the guys. Once you're on the water's edge, you can only see where you are. You can't see what's up north from the south end.'

> 'Our whole service is a bunch of surfers … If you love the water, what else do you wanna do?'

Lifeguards rotate through the three Waverley beaches on a roster system organised by Hoppo to fit the differing needs and conditions of each location. There are no women lifeguards on Waverley's roster right now; one tried out at the start of the season and passed the physicals, but didn't get a guernsey. Hoppo thinks it's a rare woman who can put up with being around so many men all the time. Maybe it's sexist, but then he has high praise for Brooke Cassell, who was a lifeguard for a couple of years in the middle of the decade and featured in the first year of the show. 'She was as good as anyone. She was small but she could get a big guy onto a board and get him in. She'd had years of experience up on the Central Coast … I think that helped her fit in.' Brooke is now an ambulance officer—a common enough career path for a highly qualified lifeguard.

Australia-wide, there might be around 500 pro lifeguards; they have an organisation (the Australian Professional Ocean Lifeguard Association, or APOLA) and a conference each year to exchange ideas and bring up issues common to all groups. The Gold Coast, the busiest single council area, probably employs 100 at peak times. 'There's a lot of phone calls in between,' says Hoppo.

'Our whole service is a bunch of surfers,' adds Kerrbox. He points to Aaron and Kobi Graham in Waverley, and Jamie Mitchell, Mick Dibetta, Michael Chan, Aaron Bitmead and Clint Robertson on the Gold Coast, as just a few examples. 'If you love the water, what else do you wanna do?'

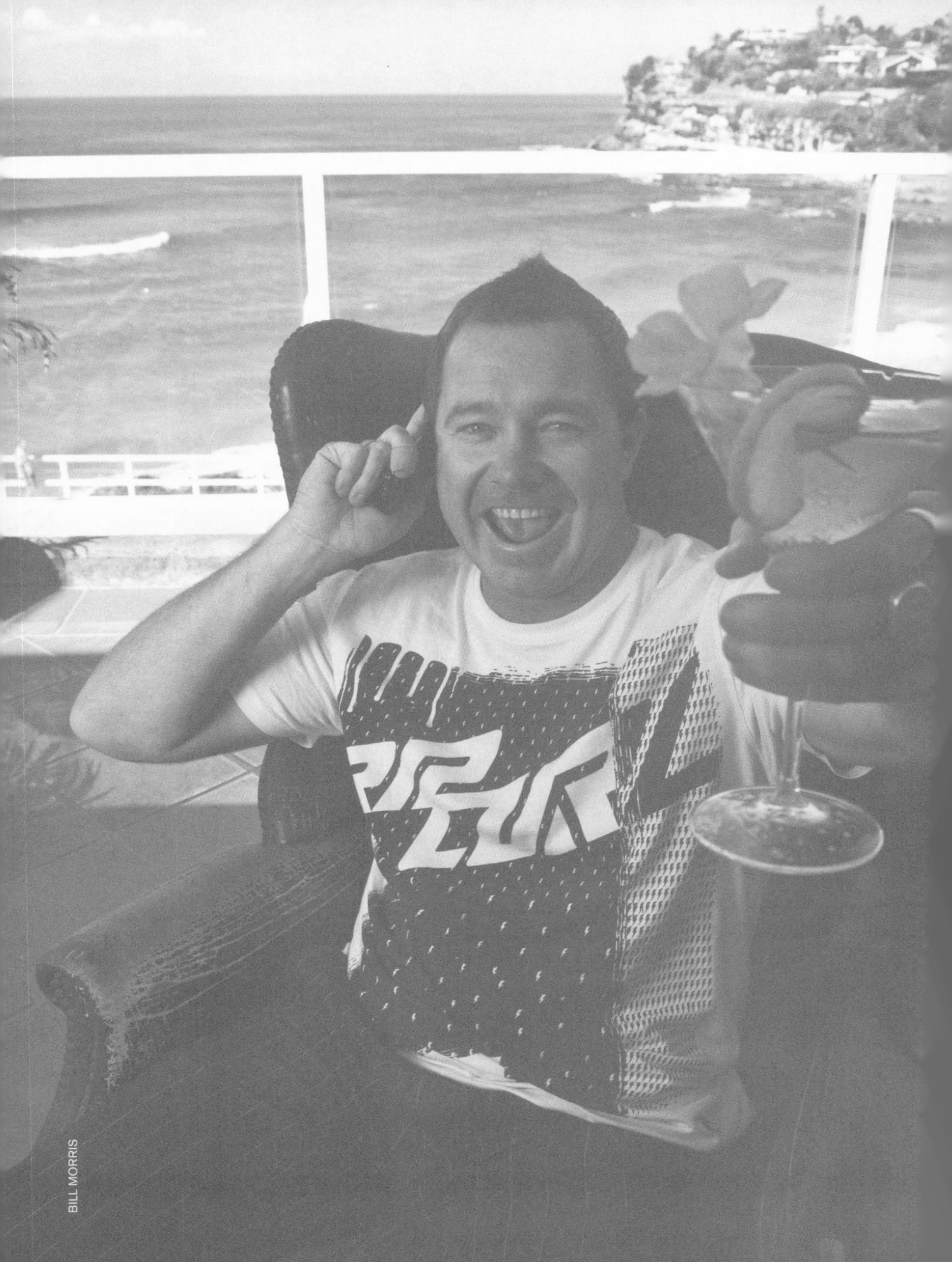

BILL MORRIS

Box: The Mascot
(Rod Kerr)

'They call me the Chosen One,' Rod Kerr says, reclining on his leather couch, with its flawless view of Bronte Beach.

Box's eyes are twinkling. Is he kidding? Heck yes, he's kidding. Making fun of stuff is one of Rodney's finely honed skills, and as becomes clear in even a short time spent in the Bondi lifeguard realm, it's something he's handed down to the crew.

Hoppo's the leader, but Kerrbox is something else, equally vital in any Aussie team—the mascot, the people's champ, simultaneously loved and mercilessly bagged by his mates. Harries calls him 'Elvis Presley, because he's the King and he lives in Graceland … He looks like Fabio and he's got Lance Armstrong's calves … no definition whatsoever.' Whippet spent several days last summer drawing tiny cartoon box heads and sticking them up around the lifeguard tower with the aid of a long pole, in places Rod couldn't possibly reach.

It hides the fact that the boys would do anything for this chunkily built, sharp-eyed former pro surfer. Rod Kerr never won a world pro title, but he made himself a pro tour legend nonetheless—

a party-lover who went out and fought like a lion for every point and made more friends than dollars. Today, he's still brightening people's lives—but in addition, he's saving them.

Rodney Graham Kerr was born on 23 July 1967, in Sydney, and still lives in the original family home, overlooking Bronte from the north. 'Best place in the whole world I think,' he says, and this time he's not making fun.

He and older sister Kathy—'We get on famously'—paid for the renovations to the place; now she lives upstairs, and Rod occupies the two-bedroom apartment downstairs. He feels like he's come out of it at the right end.

Public service—the active kind—is in Kerrbox's genes. His maternal grandfather, Todger Taylor, was a lifeguard at Tamarama, and his mum Coralie was a top swimmer. Todger was the first to put the idea of lifeguarding into Rod's head. Dad Graham grew up around Bronte, worked as a fireman for 38 years at Kings Cross station, surfed when younger, and played basketball for New South Wales, though he's no taller than Box. 'He's got a lot of good water skills though, I had him in the water yesterday and he loved it.'

Rod did Nippers with Hoppo, loved the water and the competition, then got into surfing. 'There was always a boundary between surfing and the surf clubs. But the thing was, we had nowhere else to go.'

Local surfers are a tight bunch around Bronte; Rod was invited into the boardriders' club at eleven years of age, and plunged in. By his late teens, he was on the way to a pro career. 'I played football at

RIGHT Young Rodney was a natural footballer, wreaking havoc on the field long before he did so in the water.

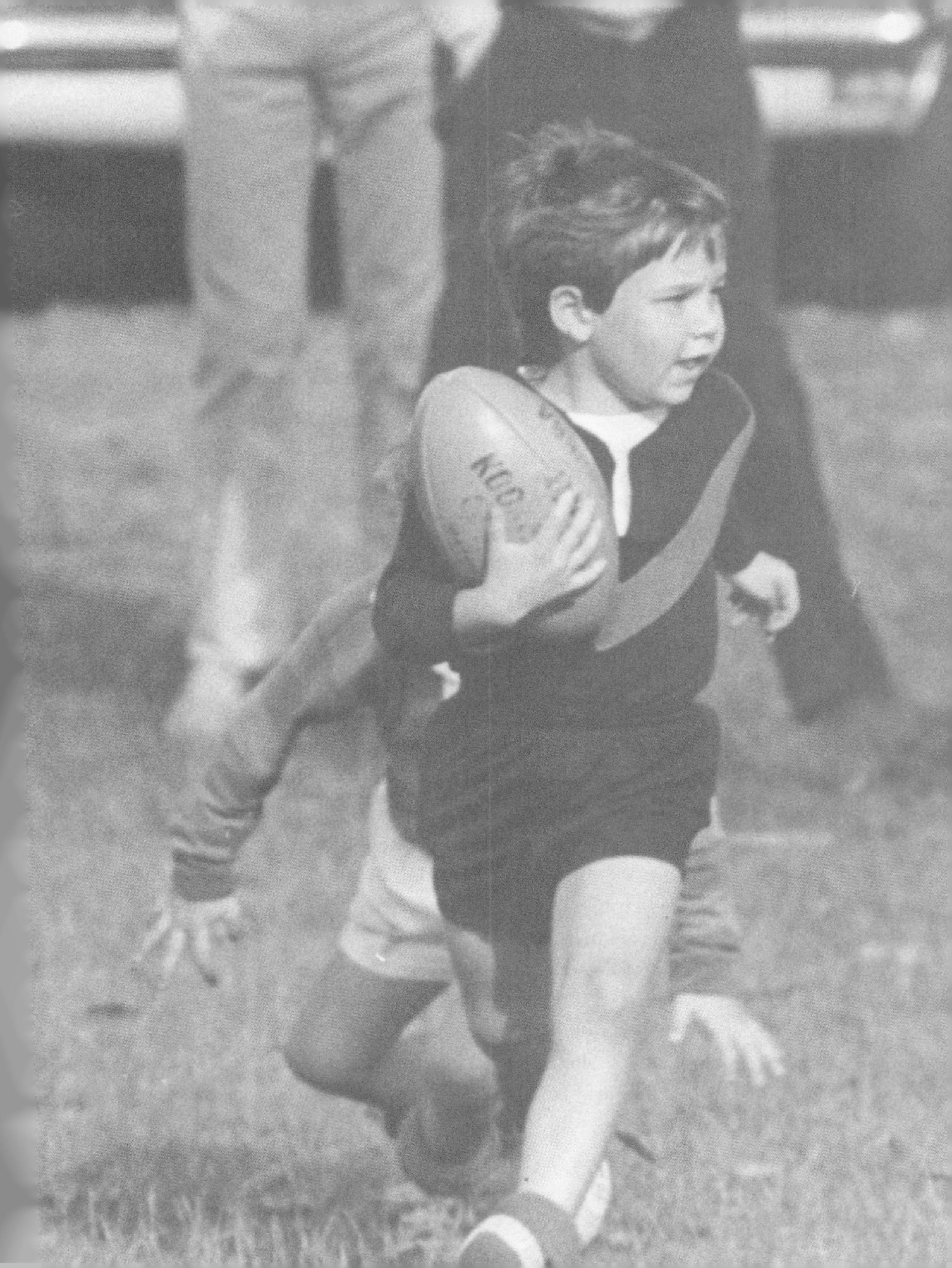

school and I was pretty good, but it was weird, I always knew I was gonna be a surfer. I don't know why I knew. I know my mum and dad spent a lot of their own money trying to get me there. But then along came Quiksilver and Rip Curl too, and things just went boom.'

'I was overwhelmed ... they said they'd love [to have] my surfing skills, but I didn't know if I could handle the blood and guts.'

He attended Marcellin College, and spearheaded their school surf team—one of the first school teams in Australia. But his last couple of school years might as well never have occurred. 'They said, "Look we know you're not gonna do your homework, you don't HAVE to, but you won't learn much." I said, "SWEET!" I'd walk into school and they'd say, "Did you do your homework?" And I'd say, "Nup." I knew straightaway I was gonna be on the tour. Couldn't wait for school to finish.'

On tour he was irrepressible. The nickname 'Kerrbox' was a gentle bagging of Hawaiian ex-pro Buzzy Kerrbox, whose name the young Aussies found inexplicably funny. Hell, everything was funny! But everything wears thin over time, and at the end of 1994 Rod flew back from Hawaii and quit, just like that. 'To tell you the truth I just missed home. All the travelling, I hated it at the end. I loved being at home.

'It was probably the hardest thing I've ever had to do. Because I didn't apply myself at school, the hard part was trying to find a job—because I had no skills. It was scary. You're thrown out there wondering what to do. As a pro I was earning five times as much as my dad. I'd be just lying around the house, and he'd be saying,

"How's this gonna work?" Now he was chuckling, going "Now you gotta get a job son!"'

He ended up repping for a clothing label for a few months, then head lifeguard George Quigley suggested he try out for the service. Hoppo, his old Nippers mate, encouraged him as well.

'I was overwhelmed, cos they'd said they would love me to be part of it with my surfing skills, but I didn't know if I could handle the other part of it, the blood and guts.' Kerrbox had three weeks to get all the certificates, and blam, suddenly he was on the beach, wondering if he could do the job at all. 'The hardest part was just turning up to work every day. Just being accountable. That was so hard. I had my first resusc six weeks into working and I was thinking, "What the fuck is going on?"'

Kerrbox lives on an emotional edge all the time; most of all he appreciates the look on people's faces when he's been able to bring them around after a near-drowning. The father of a friend has almost drowned twice—both times Box saved him. Another Bronte bloke, who's prey to anaphylaxis, Box has actually resuscitated twice. 'He looks at me and says, "Mate, I love ya." He loves me! Sickening, but it's unreal, because when you look at it, I saved his life twice! The surfing stuff's great but now it's more important what you do on the beach.'

What he still finds difficult are the long hours. Being in the sun all the time, you can get grumpy, or maybe you get a knock on the door and some lady's abusing you because there's a dog on the beach. Just the simplest things. 'The worst day is when people are being stung by bluebottles, because there's not much you can do about it and it just goes on all day. Get me outta here!'

Still, it's a vast improvement, even on fifteen years ago. 'We used to have these old hardwood red poles for flags, which I knocked

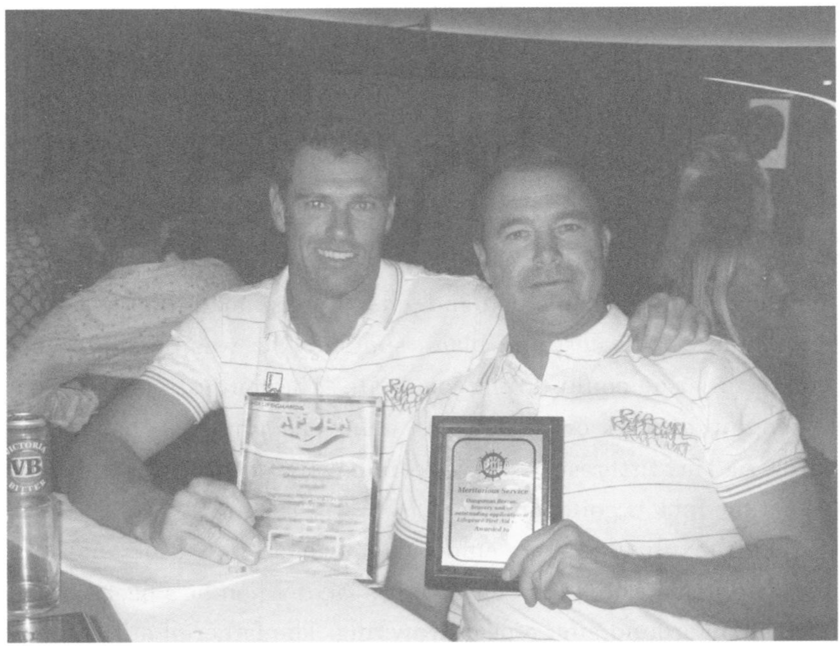

ABOVE He wins awards these days, not contests. Box with Hoppo and their APOLA commendations.

myself out with once. We had one ATV, no jet skis, no defib, the oxys were ancient … I look at it these days and go, "How did we do it?"'

He thinks the worst part was working alone. One morning early in his career, he got there to find five Japanese tourists being sucked out at the south end in heavy surf. 'It was 5 to 6 a.m. If I'd been late to work they would've been dead. I jumped in—I got four of 'em, thought I had 'em all. They were all over me, scratching me, but there was solid surf and we got washed in.

'Then I heard the crowd yelling, "There's one more! You've missed one!" This guy's face-down. I went "Oh no", bolted out and got him, swam in, started mouth-to-mouth. There was this doctor lady walking along the beach and she jumped in to help. We ended up getting him back. But from that moment on I went "That's it, I'm quitting if I have to work on my own. No way I'm doing that again".'

That day marked a change, part of the bigger change Hoppo was beginning to manage at the time: no more one-man rosters. 'My dad was stoked I got a job but I don't think hardly anybody thought what we do was a job,' says Box. 'But now it's totally different. Everyone recognises it's a real job. We're very fortunate to have a very supportive council. I think it's because the drownings don't happen anymore, they look at that and say, "Jeez, well, you guys must be doing something."

'I think we pride ourselves on what we do, we give a shit. After hours we care about what happens, and I think if we didn't we wouldn't be any good at it. You have to care.'

It kills Box when the surf is excellent, because all he can do is watch. Of the local surfers, he says: 'They're unreal. It's just the kooks. Sometimes if Tamarama is pumping, we just pull the flags down, let 'em go. But 90 per cent of the people who go surfing at Bondi, we just rat-arse 'em.'

Most scared he's been? 'I had a scare with Hoppo a couple of years ago. I had this guy, a massive Tongan, he'd gone snorkelling, for some unknown reason, and it was 8- to 10-foot surf. We jumped off the back of Bronte to get to him and we were swimming for probably 45 minutes trying to get him in. I had cuts from head to toe. I wrapped myself around him and took the hits.'

Then he describes 'the stupidest thing I've ever done as a lifeguard': 'You're supposed to radio in and tell everyone when you're going into the water, but one day I thought I was too cool for that. I went out for this guy and I was wearing a rash vest because there'd been bluebottles this day, and the guy leaped out of the water and grabbed me by the rashie and dragged me under. I thought, "Fuck, I'm gonna die here. I'm gonna drown right now." I was kicking and punching him and he wouldn't let go. I was thinking, "This is really dumb. No-one's looking, I've got nothing." Then all of a sudden he let go. One of the boys had seen what was happening and paddled out and punched the guy, knocked him out. He pulled me up by the hair and said, "You fuckin' idiot, what'd we tell you?" To this day I always tell the boys never to go out without saying so.'

> 'I think we pride ourselves on what we do ... and if we didn't we wouldn't be any good at it. You have to care.'

How long can Box go? He's been there now for fourteen years. 'I can't see myself leaving. Keeps you young, keeps you healthy, keeps you grounded. You get younger guys like Harries going, "Yeah let's go surf!" If ya don't, they rip in. They keep me young at heart and while they're doing that I'm going nowhere.' The boys respect Kerrbox but they bag him all the time, and in that classical Aussie reversal of intention, Box knows it means he's got their respect. 'I'm the first person on their list. Whippet's one of the worst, he rips in all the time, but at the end of the day I know he gives a fuck. If I wasn't there I'd be upset. If they don't bag you, you're fucked.'

His old pro surfer mates show up at Bondi from time to time—Tom Carroll, Donavon Frankenreiter, Damien Hardman, Brad Gerlach, Barton Lynch, Matt Hoy, Beau Emerton, John Shimooka,

Simon Law, Kelly Slater ... Tom especially has become friends with the boys, since his dad lives on the southern end of the beach. Box says, 'The lifeguards don't show it but they love it when the boys come down. They try to act tough but they love it!'

Like Hoppo, though, Box is beginning to suffer the slings and arrows of age. In 2008 he snapped his left Achilles tendon playing squash; it kept him out of surfing for a year. He did his first rescue a few weeks after the start of the 2009 season and he found it a scary experience. 'It's given me time to think about things,' he says. 'I've been lucky. I had two knee operations but this was a long one, and I don't think I'll ever get back to where I was, but that's cool.'

wild stories FROM THE SERVICE

The kite-surfer

KITE-SURFING IS BANNED at Bondi Beach, for a few good reasons: the craft are heavy and sharp-edged, the speeds involved are greater than anything achieved in the bay by anything but the lifeguards' jet skis, and the rigging creates dangers exaggerated by Bondi's crowds.

So when a kite-surfer unexpectedly walks down the sands and begins to kit up, the lifeguards are first surprised, then irritated. Finally they have to explain to him that there's a ban in place, which leads to an animated discussion on the beach.

'The guy was going on to us about how he was NSW kite-surfing champion,' says Kerrbox. 'We're saying it doesn't make any difference, he can't be doing it here.' Then the whole incident takes a turn for the farcical. Wind gusts keep pulling the surfer across the sand while he tries busily, then frantically, to employ a safety leash release system. It doesn't work, but the wind does; it flips the kite-surfer clean over the promenade wall and almost right into the skateboard park.

So here's how kite-surfers were banned at Bondi

ORIGINALLY THERE WAS no ban in place, and Bondi was host to a growing number of kites. But the riders would zoom up and down the beach, across flags and near groups of swimmers and surfers, so the lifeguards decided something had to be done.

They bade their time until a particularly gruesome day, when kites were coming closer than usual to other water-users, especially a group of surf-race swimmers and triathletes who were doing in-out sets in front of North Bondi surf club. When one kite strayed too close to the group, Deano, Whippet and Box decided the time had come; two of them jumped in a rhino, the other began setting up the jet ski. Just as the rhino boys took off, the kite-surfer threw caution to the winds and rode straight THROUGH the swim group. 'Whoa, buddy! In here now!' The kite-surfer came in to argue his case, but a sudden gust caught his kite and smashed him straight into the promenade.

It took the errant kiter six weeks to recover from his injuries, which weren't exactly improved when one of the near-decapitated surf swimmers showed up. 'Look away now, boys,' the swimmer told the lifeguards, before delivering his own brand of payback.

The damages claim

IT'S A SUMMER afternoon in 1997. A young man named Guy Swain comes down for a swim after a couple of beers with friends. He dives through a wave and strikes the sandbar hard with his head, suffering spinal injuries. The lifeguards treat him, call the paramedics, and Guy is off to hospital. 'We didn't hear about it again for years,' says Kerrbox. In the meantime, Mr Swain was taking Waverley Council to court, arguing that they should have warned him of the possible dangers he'd encountered to such ill effect. He won the case in front of a four-person jury in the NSW Supreme Court, then had the judgment set aside on appeal. The case then went before the High Court, and Hoppo travelled to Canberra to attend. The case revolved partly around whether the flags set-up implied some sort of negligence—that it wasn't really a safe zone as implied—and this made the lifeguards sceptical of the whole thing. 'The guy's a paraplegic, give him $10 million as far as I'm concerned,' says Box. 'Thing is he was trying to blame us. Like, it's too shallow in the flags. What, is it better if it's deep so people can drown?' But the lifeguards had no paperwork—nothing to prove exactly where they'd set the flags that afternoon, or even to show they'd recorded the incident itself. Guy Swain's High Court appeal succeeded, and the case changed almost everything about how lifeguards document their days. Since 2005 everything's recorded—every flag placement, every bit of signage, every incident—and Hoppo's got to admit it's been of benefit. 'There's a lot more paperwork generally now,' he says. 'But we can go to a computer now and trace everything precisely. Years down the line we can pull up a day and tell you exactly where we set up the beach and what happened. It's part of the professionalism we've been working on.'

The seal that got away

WANT TO KNOCK a lifeguard out? This story should give you a few clues. One winter morning, Harries and Box are on duty when two girls come up to report a seal. 'We saw it go up the big drainage pipe at the end of the beach,' they tell the boys. Kerrbox doesn't really believe it—there are 40 metres of sharp rock between the water and the pipe—but the guards have to do something. 'So off we go, two brave hunters with our torches, followed by these two girls, and we climb down this pipe,' recounts Box, trying not to burst out laughing. The drainpipe narrows for some distance, about 100 metres, until it splits into two separate pipes, each about a metre across. At this point, the pair are amazed to find the seal, crouched near the entrance to one of the tunnels. It snorts angrily at them. The brave hunters decide to seek a second opinion, so they retreat to the tower and call Taronga Zoo, which counsels them to leave it alone for now. Next morning nobody's sure what's happened to the seal, and the zoo advises the lifeguards to do a check and make sure nothing's gone wrong. So down they go again, check the tunnel, and no seal. Box turns to head back, when suddenly there's a SPLAT! and the enraged seal comes charging out of the OTHER tunnel! It'd been lying in wait. 'It outsmarted us,' says Box. 'I just took off, running my guts out and not thinking of anything but getting away from this pissed-off seal, and I ran clean into the lip of the pipe with my head. Knocked me flat on my back.' Sadly there is no film of this event. The seal got away.

8 TOP Pieces of gear

Aside from their water skills and five senses, here's what the boys most need in order to do their job:

1. Radio

Communication's at the top of the list for any lifeguard team; everyone who leaves the tower carries one, putting them in instant touch with each other and with whoever's got the control point in the tower itself. 'It promotes teamwork,' says Hoppo. 'And it can be a lifeline for a stranded team member.'

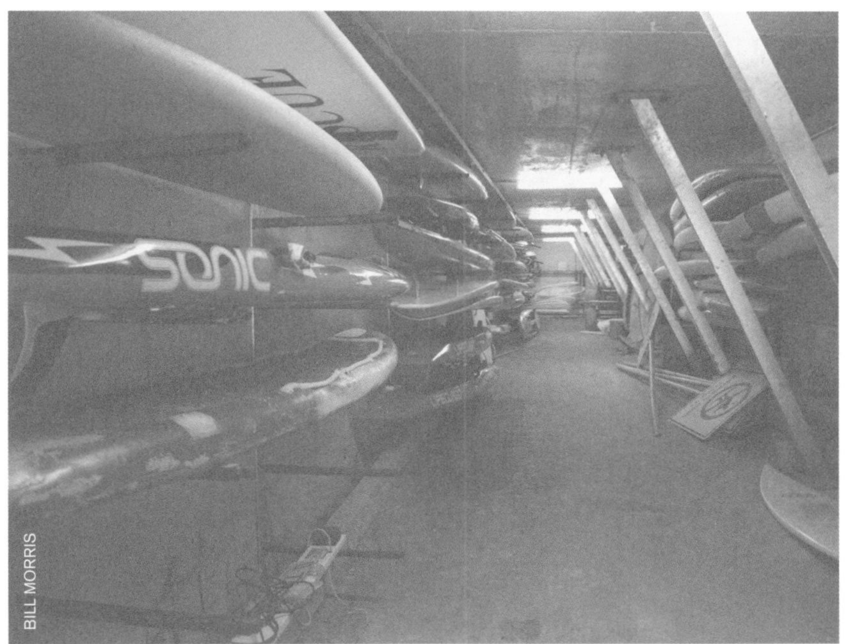

BILL MORRIS

2. Board

The rescue board, all 2.8 metres and 12 kilos of it, is the craft of first resort in almost every situation. Partly this is because they're so handy: Boards are set up at key spots along the beach, and one's strapped to every ATV, so they're immediately available to a roaming lifeguard. But partly it's because the boys are surfers by instinct; without exception they can handle the board superbly.

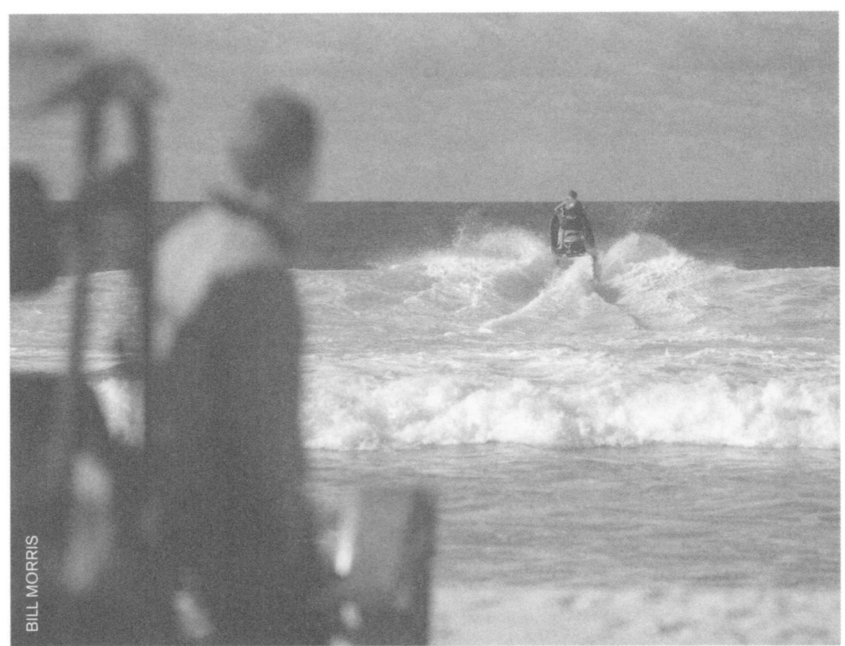
BILL MORRIS

3. Jet ski

Once it's in the water, the ski is the ultimate rescue device: fast, able to cope with any surf and support a number of patients in a pinch. It has another, less obvious value: Lifeguards don't exhaust themselves while using it, the way they do on a board or while·swimming. 'On busy days it keeps the physical workload low and the energy levels high,' says Tom.

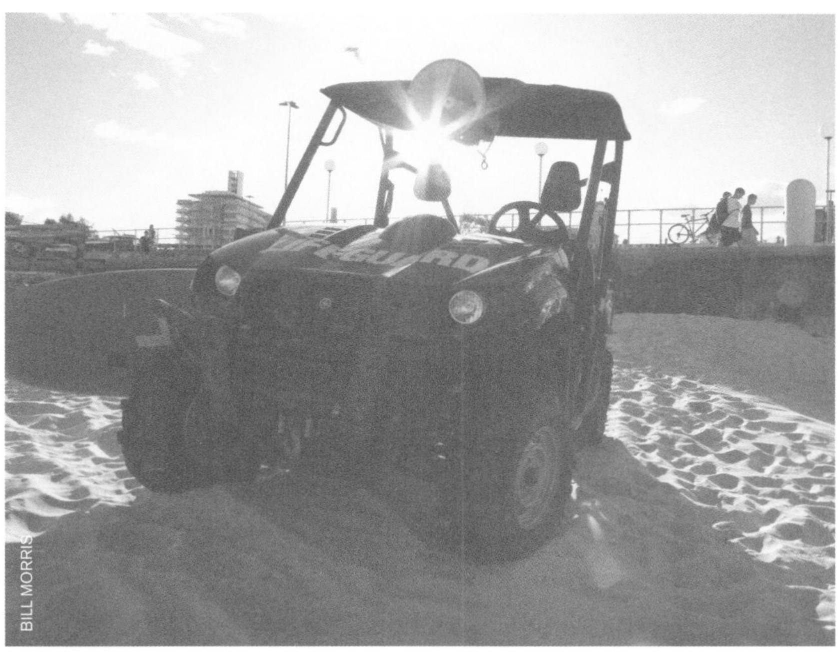

BILL MORRIS

4. The ATVs, or 'rhinos'

These little workhorses are all about swift access. They can carry lifeguards, boards, defibrillators, oxygen and spinal boards to the water's edge, and patients back, far faster than anyone can run. At another level, they're a strong reminder of the lifeguard presence–a kind of roving tower. At still another, they'll carry a lot of flags and signs at the end of a busy day.

5. Megaphone

Again, communication, though this time it's with the customers. The rhinos carry one of these per vehicle; the boys can use them to talk swimmers and surfers through an encounter with a rip or other sticky situation. 'We prevent a lot of rescues that way,' says Deano. 'It saves us a lot of water time.'

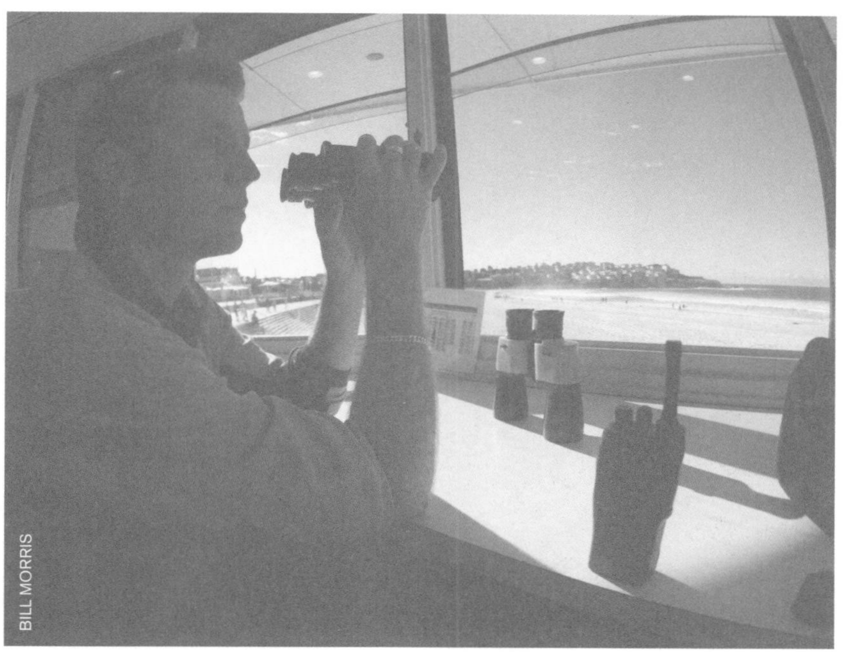

BILL MORRIS

6. Binoculars

Another way of covering ground fast. From the tower, binoculars give a lifeguard visual access to the potentially lethal south-end channels and rips, and to the water outside the break … not to mention tracking thieves through the mid-Bondi crowds.

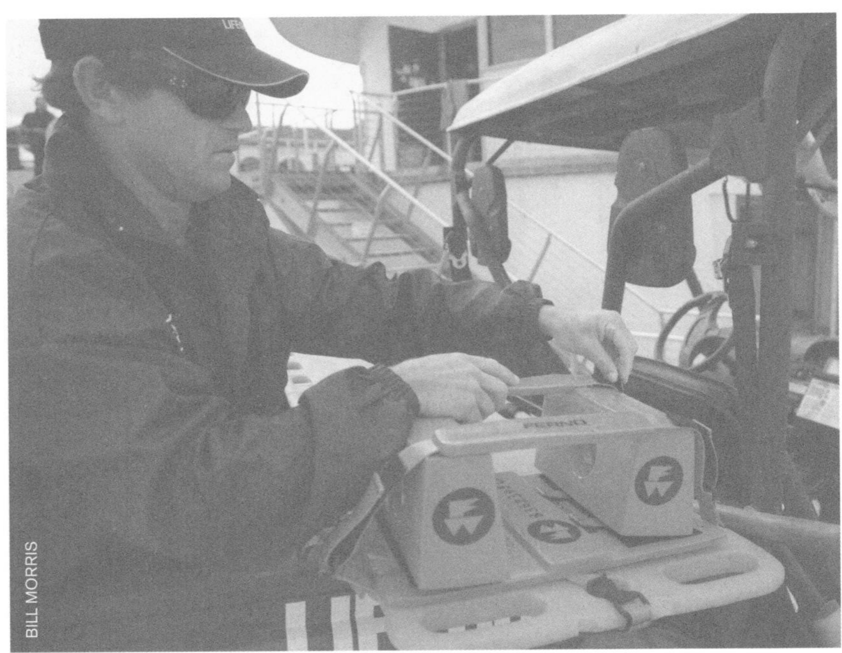
BILL MORRIS

7. Defibrillator

Portable and quickly deployed by any trained lifeguard, it does the big job in any critical resuscitation: it tracks the patient's heartbeat (or lack of), informs the team, and delivers a heart-starting electric shock if needed.

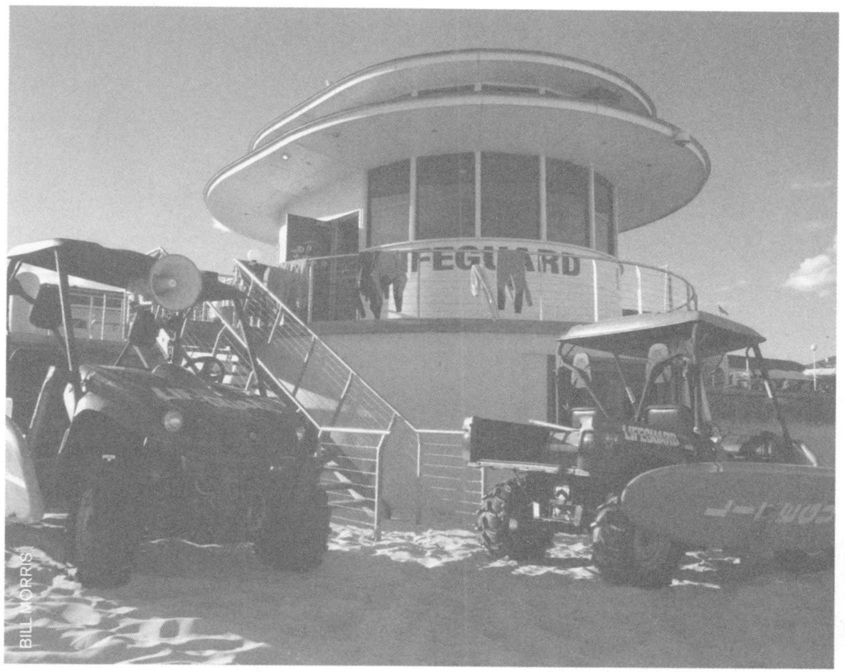

BILL MORRIS

8. The key to the tower's front door

'Sounds funny on a list like this,' says Harries, 'but if you can't get in, then you can't use any of the gear. And forgetting the key–it's a classic rookie mistake. Someone always gets caught out.'

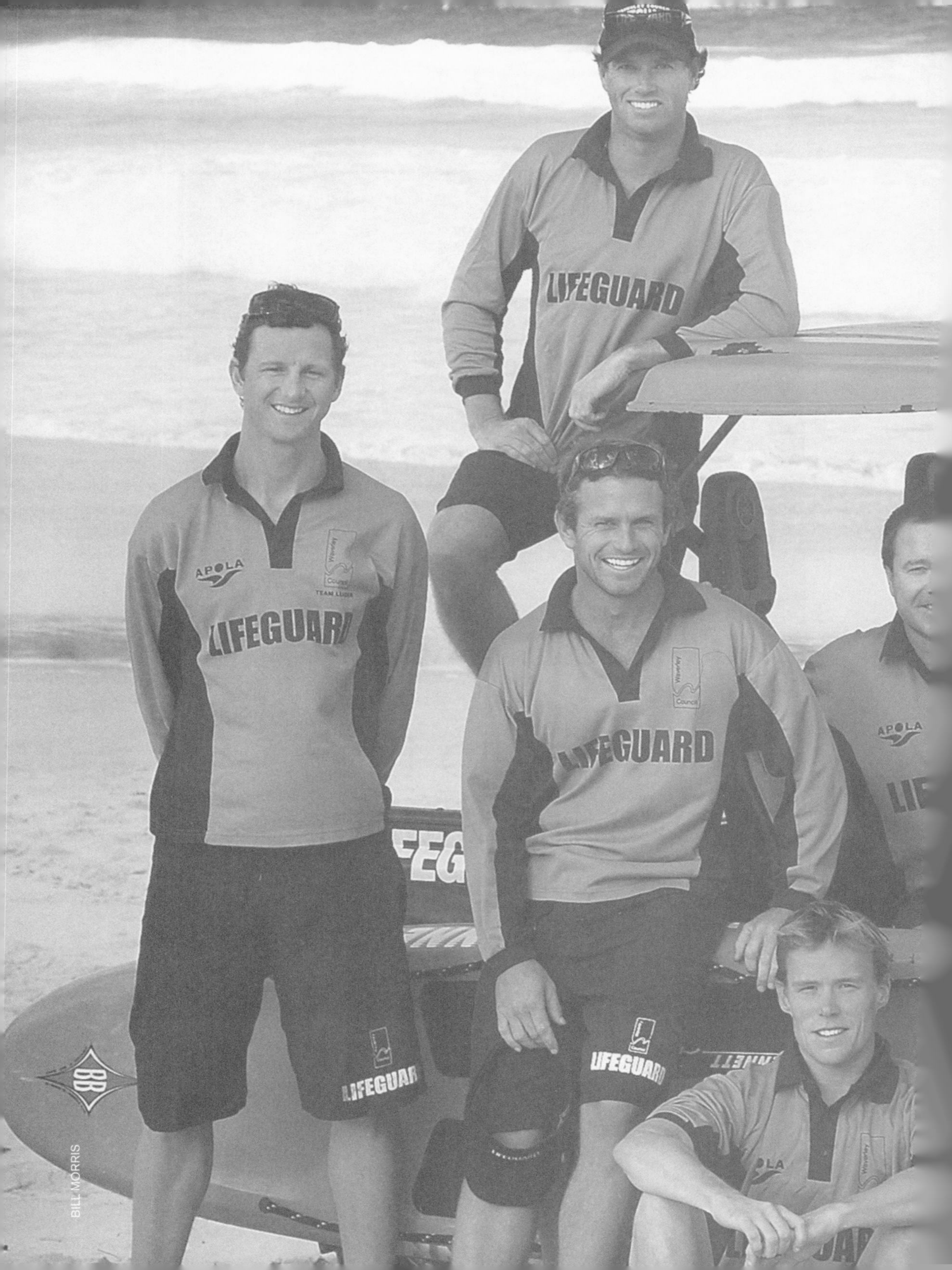

BILL MORRIS

3
THE SHOW

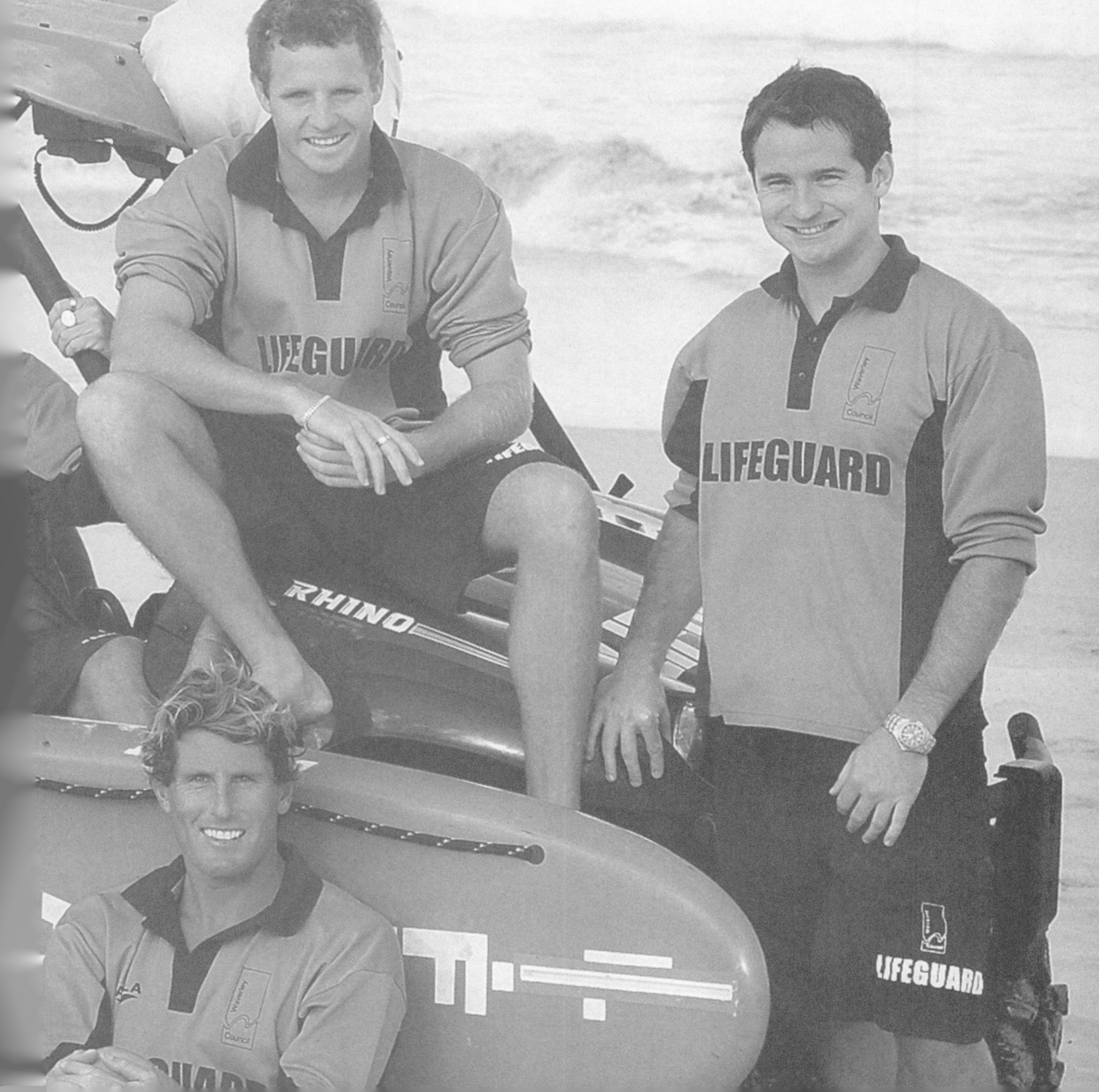

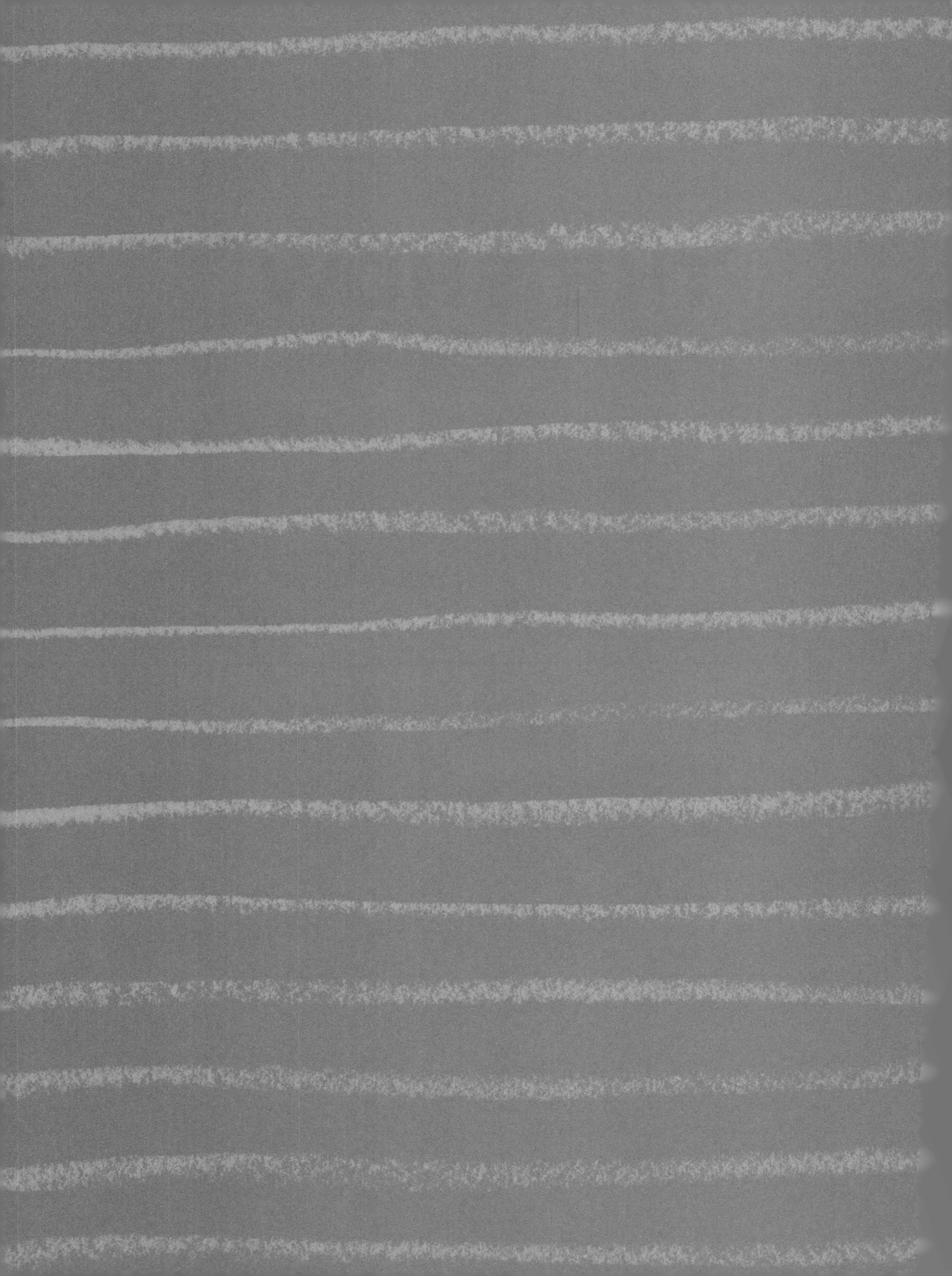

How a hit TV series rose out of the Bondi waves

In the era of documentary television, it's a slam dunk—girls, sun, iconic beach culture ... and danger, even tragedy, lurking in the background. Yet the *Bondi Rescue* show relied for its inception on a chance job offer and a hopeful local boy. The rest? Put it down to the beach—and a lot of damn hard work.

Ben Davies is the guy who had the initial idea for a show based on the Bondi lifeguard service. Meet him at the lifeguard tower on a weekday afternoon, and whatever your image is of a Sydney eastern suburbs 'TV producer'—Glossy? Snappy dresser? Bullshit artist?—it'll almost certainly be dispelled. Ben, now 37 years of age, is an original Bondi boy, rugged-faced and fit, who went to a local school (Waverley College), played footy (Bondi United), and was president of the local boardriders' club. Like a lot of the lifeguards, he has a vaguely old-fashioned feel about him, a reminder of the area's working-class days. 'Product of the Bondi institutions, I s'pose you could say,' he grins.

Intrigued by film and TV, he finished uni then dived in head-first by entering the ABC's Race Around The World competition for young film-makers. By 2004, he'd come home from a trip overseas and was holed up in an apartment across the road from the beach, fuelled by a writer's development grant, and tapping away on his computer, and he admits, 'I was kinda making very slow progress there. I was going a bit stir-crazy up in my room staring at the laptop. A couple of the boys said to me, "Come and work on the beach." I thought it'd be a good idea, bring a couple of extra dollars in.'

The lifeguard service had a mid-year intake to supplement numbers, so Ben hopped in, did the tests, and started on New Year's Eve 2004. The day blew his mind: 'The beach was absolutely throbbing with people and going bananas, and I thought, "This is insane!" After living and surfing here all my life, I never knew what went on in the job. I always had high regard for the lifeguards but I thought they were really just having a good time, taking off their shirts and talking to girls, all that jazz. I was amazed by the stuff that happened.' Immediately he knew there was an idea here for a TV project.

Davies had been thinking about the show for a year, but when Channel Ten pressed the buzzer, he was hurled into fast-forward.

Ben started with Dave Gyngell, the local Bondi surfer who'd gained a lot of traction in the TV industry and who helped drive the idea along to the point where a production company was needed. Next stop was Michael Cordell, a highly experienced independent producer who'd given Ben work in the past. 'I kinda knew it was a bit of a no-brainer. Michael said righto and cut a deal and we went hunting a broadcaster.' They had a funny reaction from the broadcasters at first—even from their future home at Channel Ten. People would say what Ben himself had assumed: 'I go down to

Bondi and there's not that much happening down there.' In fact the summer of 2004–05 had been ultra dramatic, with twelve critical resuscitations and many more incidents. In a way it's the *Bondi Rescue* year that should've been.

For the 2005–06 summer, through the very supportive David Mott, Ten agreed to a single pilot show, but then the beach became a newly dramatic focus of attention. 'There were the Cronulla riots, there were sharks, and heatwaves, all this kind of stuff happening in beach culture, and they said "OK, let's make a series".'

Few people watching a TV show have any idea of the crazy stresses and workloads involved—especially surrounding an untested concept. Ben had been thinking about it for a year, but when the buzzer sounded, he was hurled into fast-forward. 'It sounds easier than it was. It freaked me out actually. We didn't get the go-ahead until two weeks before. We had two weeks to hire everyone and work it all out … and it worked out—just.'

Ben never considered including the local surf clubs. The SLSA has had an uncertain relationship with the show; at first they didn't want to be part of it, then they did, then they told the Bondi surf club members they couldn't be part of it. 'I've got affection for the clubs and a lot of my mates are still in 'em, but I knew the volume of activity was happening with the professional lifeguards. They're the ones who have the duty of care on the beach.'

The crew learned on the job. First lesson: don't run around like chooks with their heads cut off. 'In the beginning I thought we had to film everything—everything was a story, you know. Plus we didn't have the technology we have now. The stories weren't being covered as well as they are today … we were pinballing from one thing to another, it was overwhelming. But really it's taken an organic course through a lot of trial and error.'

At first he didn't realise how important the lifeguards themselves would be, expecting the drama of the situations to carry the show. But when he was back in the editing bay watching the rushes, Ben began to see how vital the characters were. Viewers would care about the drama, because the guys encountering it were loveable. 'They were really appealing Australian characters. I was saying to people at that point, "There's the gauchos in Argentina and the Alpine Patrol in the Swiss Alps, but Australia's got its lifeguards", and these guys reflected that. In a way they're archetypes.'

Plus it cast an entirely new light on Bondi—this beach everyone thought they knew, but didn't at all.

Ben's learning curves never stopped. He frames the essentials of the show quite simply: 'Stuff just happens and all of a sudden it's HAPPENING. It's not like a police show where you hear something's happening over the radio then you arrive and it's already happened and the situation has changed. Here there's no beginning, all of a sudden someone's drowning and everything starts there. So that was kinda weird, there's no empathy for the character, it's just a head going underwater.' Typically a *Bondi Rescue* piece starts that way—a blank slate, the story only unravelling once the victim is back on the beach and safe, talking with the lifeguard, often still in minor shock at having avoided death by a matter of minutes or seconds.

This means a lot of weight rests on the portrayal of the rescue itself, something Ben feels they're only just starting to capture now after four seasons. 'I think I've only seen one rescue which shows what it's really like to DO a rescue … and we've shot thousands of rescues. The cameras on the boards, the long-range up in the tower, the microphones in the water. We have all these things to help you get a sense of it. The first series we just shot from the beach, the guys just disappeared out to sea and brought 'em in. I remember the first time we used a water mic, the first guy who had one on paddled out and said to the patient, "G'day, how are you, are you alright?" Then he said, "Where are you from?" They were paddling in, having this boring sort of conversation, and we were up in the tower with headsets on, just riveted! It was like a whole new world.'

Getting inside the rescue is the big one. But there's tracking it all along, watching the lifeguards themselves dealing with the season, facing their own challenges, some they've set for themselves and some coming as a surprise.

Of which the series itself has been the biggest. *Bondi Rescue* is a case study in the famous Uncertainty Principle: observing the lifeguards has effectively changed the job. Fame works in different ways for different people, and for many of these young men, it's been a phenomenally weird, exciting, even scary experience. For one thing, they've had to grow used to working in a fish-bowl. Ben has noticed a kind of anxiety surfacing at times: 'You don't want to be the one who misses something. It's made everyone a lot more vigilant, because they know if they bugger it up they're gonna get caught out on camera.'

On *Bondi Rescue*, 'stuff just happens and all of a sudden it's HAPPENING. There's no beginning. All of a sudden someone's drowning.'

It's also upped the ante on the Lifeguard Challenge. Once a semi-casual fitness exercise, this run–swim–board paddle from Bondi to Bronte and back has evolved into a full-on race for which the boys train like animals. 'Before the series started,' says Ben, 'we just took off together and did it and if we were getting close to the end people would wait for each other. Now they're just smashing each other. It's a lot more competitive.'

The guards have a range of views on the series' effects. Whippet and Reidy think it's reducing the rescue rate, because people are paying the flags and signs more attention. Kerrbox thinks people are more needy, looking for help more often for simple things like sunburn and bluebottle stings. Hoppo's thankful for the professional recognition; Harries loves the spotlight; Corey thinks it's funny that some viewers think the rescues are acted (they're not—among other things, there's no need). Deano just tries to get the job done. Tom wonders what will happen after the show's time has passed and some of its glamour fades from their work—will everyone stick around, or will some go downhill, like pro athletes who're past their competitive days?

While the lifeguards are sometimes the butt of each others' jokes, the patients themselves are never made fun of.

For all of them, though, Bondi is a lot more than a film set. Ben makes the point that everyone in the service has a long family association with the area, and he thinks the people who most appreciate the show are people from a similar background—long-term locals who tell him they really like the show and what it's done for the lifeguards. 'You can see the boys have got a sense of custodianship, they want people to come to the area and have a good time. They don't like to see people coming down and causing trouble, and they don't like seeing people get in trouble in the water. They like to see everyone go home safely and feeling like the beach was a good place to be.'

The lifeguards' ability to anticipate problems has paid off for the show, because it gives the TV crew time to get in position before a rescue needs to happen. This is why some of the rescues seem almost set pieces.

A typical *Bondi Rescue* crew is twelve people: a water camera, two land cameras, two sound, two field producers, two production assistants, a tower director, Ben, and a driver. Sometimes a third camera crew is thrown in on busy days. There's at least one crew on Bondi from 9 a.m. to 7 p.m. every day from mid-December till the end of March; fortunately they and the lifeguards get on well, though once the filming season's over and the cameras have gone, you can feel a palpable lessening of tension in the tower.

Often Ben's there himself, but not all the time, not anymore. 'In the beginning I went five months being here every day, living and breathing it. It was my big break, you know, I was a young field producer wanting to make it to being a producer myself, and I just went, "I'm not gonna fuck this up. I don't want to blow it",' he says, sounding rather like his lifeguard subjects when faced with a big rescue. He'd be on the shoot all day, back in the edit suite till midnight, then be on the beach again at 6 a.m. 'It's still almost six days a week.'

The show does something quite tricky and, it has to be said, unusual for a factual TV series: It somehow avoids any sense of exploitation. While the lifeguards are sometimes the butt of each other's jokes, the patients are never made fun of. This is quite conscious on Ben's part; like a lot of surfers, he puts a fair bit of emphasis on the word 'respect'. He says, 'Sometimes there can be a temptation to put a spin on things, but I think more often than not it'll come back and bite you on the bum. It's just usually better to treat people fairly and decently and they'll respond in the same way.' Stories have been pulled as a result of this thinking, at least once within hours of going to air. Like the time during this season when a kid with epilepsy had been rescued. It was a great story, but when the kid asked for it not to be shown, Ben pulled it without question.

Of course if there's no respect shown in the first place, it can work differently. The infamous kite-surfer was an example. Ben says, 'He knew there was no kite-surfing allowed at Bondi, and he rang and said "I don't want to be on, blah blah blah", and I told him, "You knew kite-surfing was banned here, you knew we were filming, I'm gonna run it. Too bad".'

High point ratings? In 2007 *Bondi Rescue* hit a peak of 1.7 million viewers with a big episode, and averaged around 1.37 million. Next season they had a lot stiffer competition, yet still managed ratings beyond 1.5 million. Ben explains: 'People will tune in for different things—we had an episode recently with a dead body retrieval, a lot of people wanted to see that. We don't sensationalise things so it's a fine line ... I think because we don't sensationalise, we're not like the boy who cried wolf—people will go along with us. Maybe if we know it's gonna be the last episode ever, we might wave the flag a bit!'

Bondi Rescue Bali was Ben's idea—a way to extend the franchise through winter. It was another last-minute effort: 'We got over there OK and did the series, but it just didn't rate. [Another show] was going full steam ahead and it ate up our target audience and we got pulled. Not the desired result,' he says wryly. The best Bali episodes remain unseen—they may still go to air. One thing Ben thinks of as an achievement was the lifeguards' donation of $25,000 to the Kuta Beach guards, which bought boards, an ATV, and resuscitation equipment. 'That gear's already saved lives, so we think it was worth it just on that basis.'

What ground remains to be covered? Ben knows some of it at least relies on the show's biggest star: Bondi herself. 'I think it's up to the beach really. And the new guys who come on, the relationships between them and the way lives change over the summers. There might be one more series, there might be five. More than anything it's up to the audience. It's commercial TV, if they keep watching 'em we'll keep making 'em. I don't want to be in the situation when dwindling ratings force us to introduce stupid crap. We don't want to jump the shark.'

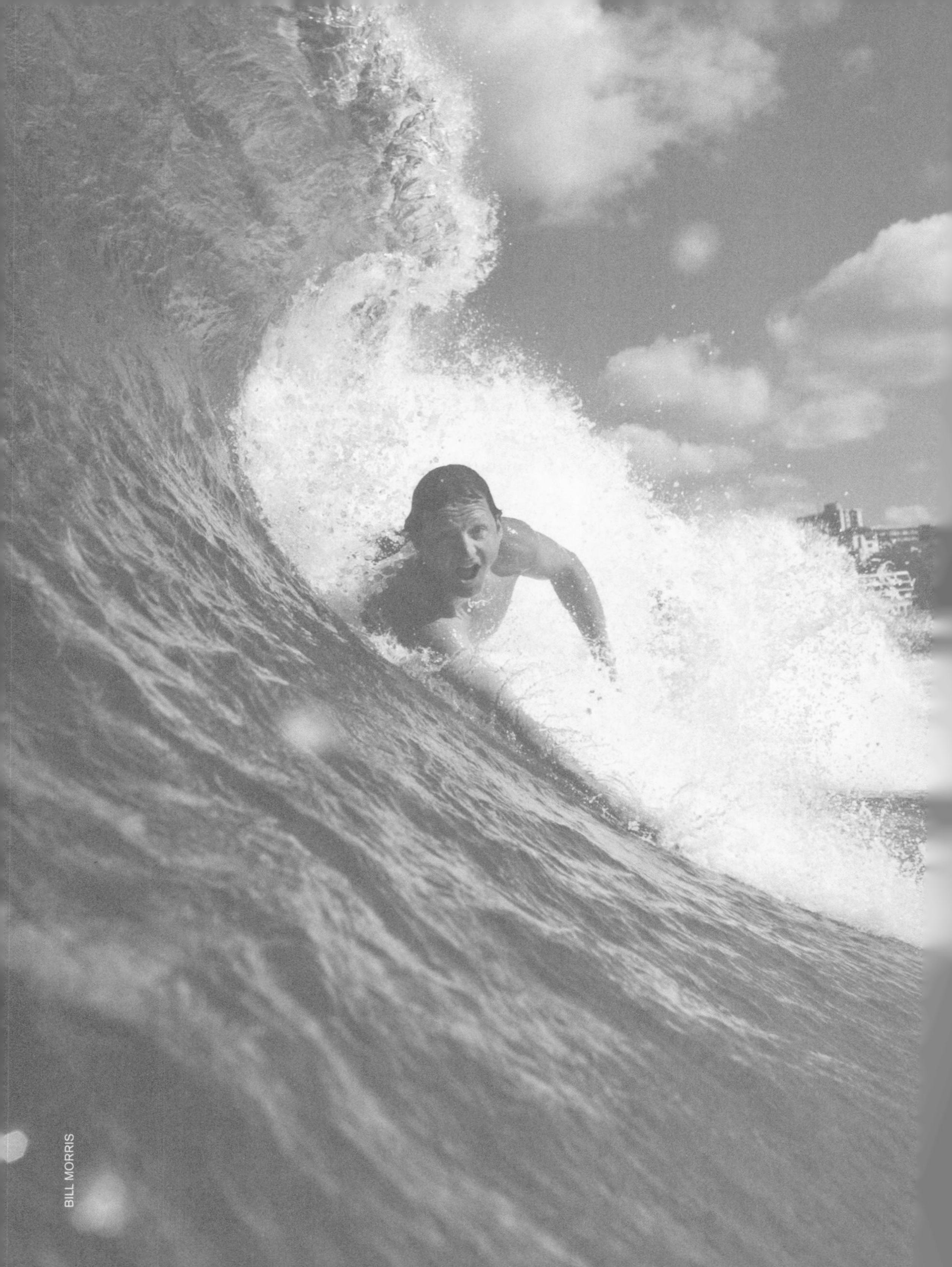

BILL MORRIS

Deano: The Swimmer
(Dean Gladstone)

It's just as well the ceilings in Dean Gladstone's place are classically high-set—because Deano is tall. Really tall. The fastest swimmer in the *Bondi Rescue* crew towers over his visitor like a genial Coogee Beach version of Grant Hackett, offering water, tea and a seat near the window—in what seems like the nice roomy flat's smallest possible space. 'Yeah, there's a bit of room,' he says, somehow managing not to use it all up with his stretched-out arms and legs. For a tall bloke, he manages to fit in surprisingly well.

Dean's local-beach roots run deep as he is tall. This apartment, where he lives with his wife Lily within a quick run of Coogee, once belonged to his grandmother. His parents have given the couple a year of rent-free living while they save for a house and prepare to put down roots of their own.

Quiet, humble and relaxed, Dean is a foil to Harries and Box with their sharp wit and exuberance. He was one of Hoppo's 'turnaround' recruits, hired into the lifeguard service at the end of 2000 as part of the new blood—the committed water-boys who revitalised the service. Now Deano is one of the leaders himself, and, he says, 'I'm starting to think we're the new old guard.'

Dean Andrew Gladstone was born on 15 September 1978, and grew up in the family home at Matraville, before the Gladstones moved to Maroubra when Dean was thirteen. There's a younger sister, Belinda; she and Dean were always close, and they had to be, they spent so much time together at swim squad and in the Coogee Surf Club Nippers. They were full-on Aussie water-kids. 'We were in the pool at home or at swimming training, if we weren't at swimming training we were at the beach.'

Belinda swam Olympic qualifying times and went on to become one of Australia's champion ironwoman racers, while laidback Dean ended up at Maroubra surf club with some mates. He regarded himself as 'lazy' because he didn't overtrain, but seemed to win swim races anyway—four silver medals and a bronze at the Australian surf lifesaving championships, in fact, doing taplin teams and surf races. He still gets goosebumps thinking about it—the adrenaline, the intensity of racing.

Eventually he quit around 2004, partly because of his life-guarding career. 'I was spending too much time at the beach. Plus because I was doing the early shift, I couldn't do swimming training.' As anyone who's done it knows, there's no racing without training.

Their dad, Daniel, was athletically inclined, a former footballer who surfed years ago and still owns a couple of boards. Mum Joanne is a nurse, and 'not the athletic type', according to Dean. Daniel and Joanne split eight years ago. 'Mum was pregnant with me at her 21st

RIGHT The water is Deano's second home. Outside the south end, May 2009.

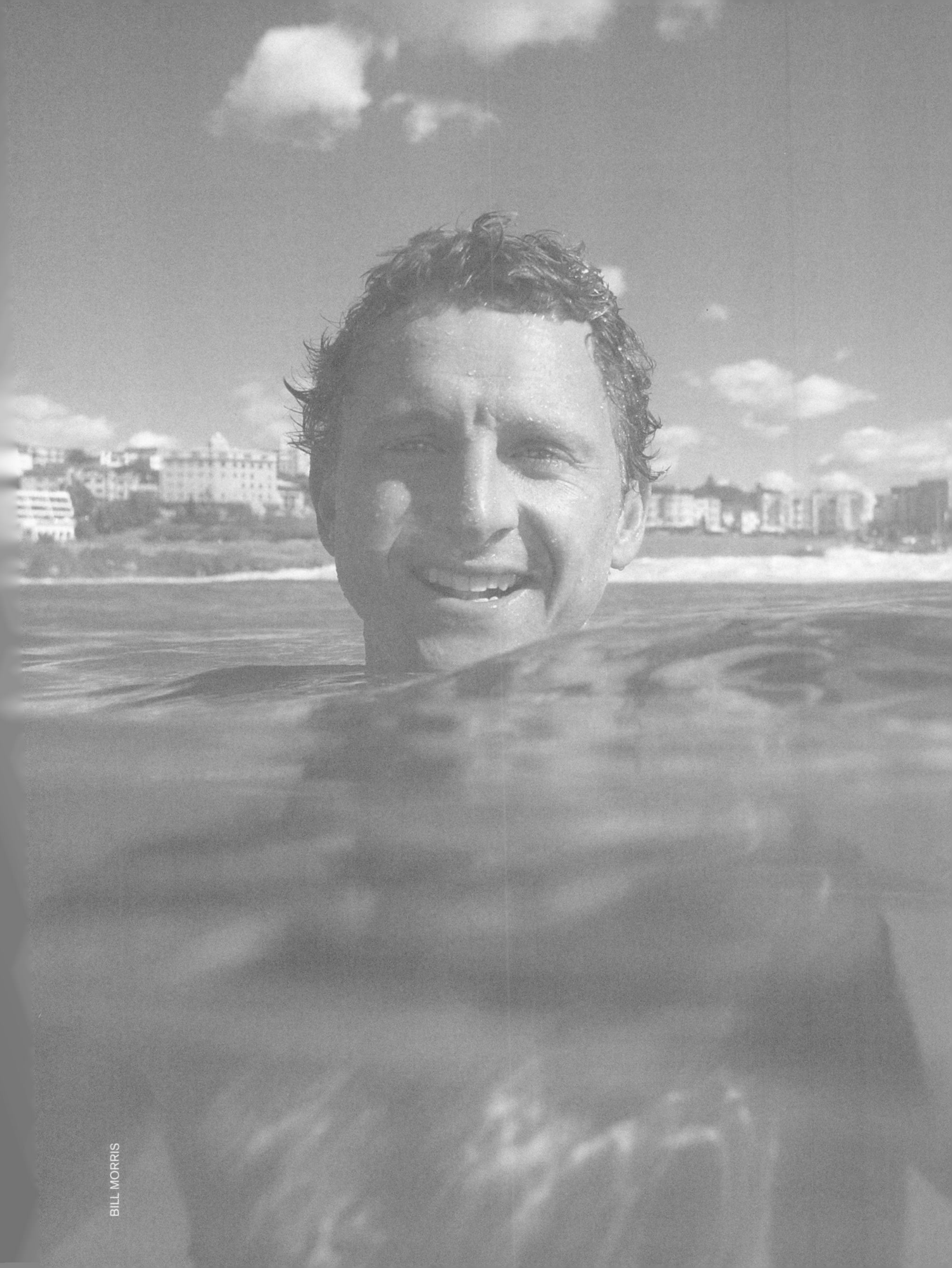

BILL MORRIS

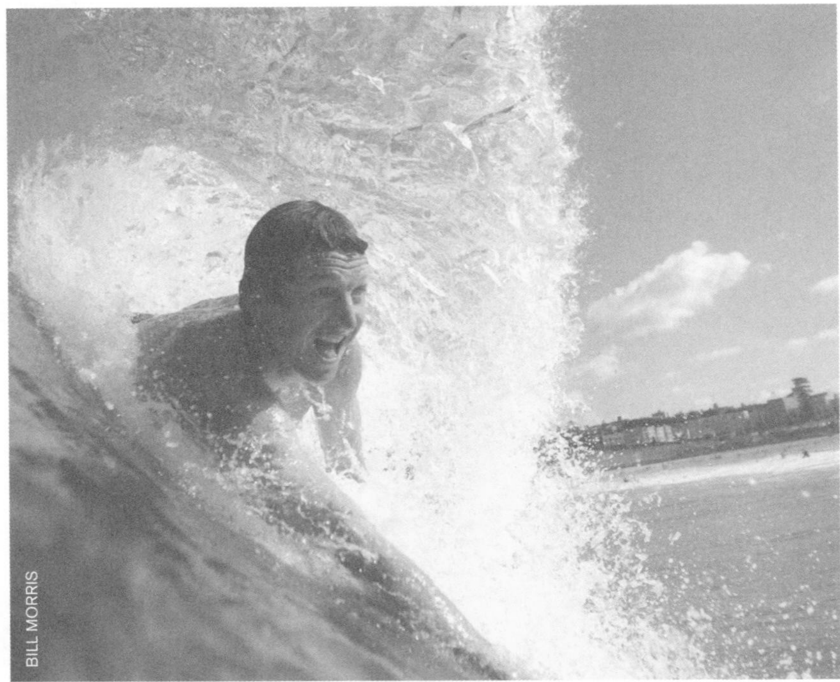

BILL MORRIS

ABOVE 'If we weren't at swimming training, we were at the beach.'

birthday party, so they were pretty young ... She worked a lot of night duties when we were growing up. She used to drop us at school at 9 a.m. and pick us up at 3.30. How did she do it? I guess parents just do it, don't they?'

Deano finished Year 12 at Marist College Pagewood, but says he didn't learn much—something he discovered later as an apprentice plumber trying to read street directories. His sister, now an occupational therapist, suspects he might have been dyslexic. 'Belinda left there and went to a public school and loved it! It was what I'd have liked to do. I kinda regret some of that now. When they shove a microphone in your face, it'd be nice to say something a bit better, or write emails a bit better, especially for work.'

Dean is too modest about his communication skills. In a social setting, surrounded by his raucous fellow lifeguards, he hangs back and doesn't say much, and the impression is of someone who's shy and unsure of himself. By himself, one-on-one, he's very different. He watches you closely through opaque blue eyes, smiles easily, speaks directly, and doesn't always say what you're expecting to hear. There's not much spin with Dean.

Later, at work, he tells a story that explains a little more about his seemingly quiet nature. In 2002 he was inadvertently involved in a dispute between a close relative and another local family. Years later, in 2005, Dean was sitting at the footy—a Roosters game of course—when a member of the disputing family came running up out of the blue and king-hit him, knocking out all his front teeth and leaving him with serious chronic health problems, including neck and shoulder pain, loss of appetite, nausea and depression.

'People ask if it's safe to swim out there. I tell 'em it's a double-ended question, I don't know if you can swim or not.'

'I was lucky to have all these blokes down here to support me,' Deano says, meaning his fellow lifeguards. 'I don't know what I would have done. I couldn't swim hard because it just hurt the neck too much. It really got me down. I trained hard this year and it was good to feel it coming back.' But he still can't enjoy a beer the way he did. The ensuing court case was settled only this season.

Dean isn't a hardcore surfer in the mould of Harries or Box or Whippet. He bodyboarded till he was thirteen, and then began to surf a lot with some of the Maroubra crew, but didn't really relish that crews' love of a blue. 'I'm not a fighter,' he says, a comment tinged with irony, given recent events. But he was always happy to go out in bigger surf, confident of himself after all those pool squads and Nipper races.

Maybe because of his dyslexia, maybe because of his own extraordinary swimming and surf skills, Dean tends to prize those skills in his fellow lifeguards. 'The best lifeguards are the best surfers. Straight up. I've spent a considerable amount of time in the ocean, I'm one of the best swimmers down there, so that qualifies me a bit, but without the surfing ability … no.'

How does Bondi fit into his picture of the eastern beaches? 'Bondi's always a bit further away for me. I didn't spend much time there as a kid. It was always the trendy place. I didn't surf there much, thought there was smaller waves, there probably is in summer. Then in winter southerly swells get really big. There's always potential to be dangerous. People go, "Is it safe to swim out there?" I say, "Well, it's a double-ended question that one, how long's a piece of string? I don't know if you can swim or not." We have busy days when it's 2 feet.'

Dean has a dry yet realistic picture of many of the rescues they perform on those small-surf days: 'The surf's not big and rough and they're not far offshore, and they've just slipped off a sandbank and exerted themselves enough to get tired. We've got nice big boards and it's easy to get two people onto 'em and catch a wave in. They get a buzz from it half the time. You have to let 'em know how much trouble they could have been in sometimes.

deano the swimmer

'You see people drowning where they can almost stand up.'

One of a lifeguard's hidden enemies is frustration. At Bondi, where people often jump straight back into the rip they've just been dragged out of, even the patience of a Dean will be tested. He believes that 'some people need to be yelled at', but he's aware of the need to let go. 'When we get out there sometimes people say they're alright, and we go "Sure", and just hang around and wait till they're in trouble. You know how Harries is always happy? Well, we just try and enjoy the job now. Don't take anything personally. If they say "Piss off", just say "Sweet! Have a good day!" And leave 'em alone, you know?'

His worst day was an Easter Monday a few years back, during a massive cyclone swell. Dean was doing a rescue in the north corner and noticed a bunch of people being swept out near the central flags. 'There were about six people in trouble. I left four with the board and swam over and pulled the other two up. Later someone came and said, "We're missing a friend." So we got serious. Got the helicopter in. But he never ever showed up. Some of the boys were saying it might be a bit of a fake-your-own-death-and-stay-in-Australia thing, but it was pretty believable.'

'You see people drowning where they can almost stand up.'

Dean did SLSC patrols at Coogee and Maroubra for around ten years, which gives him an insider's take on the difference between volunteers and pros. 'I did most of my patrolling before I was a lifeguard, so, as a volunteer, you're just not aware of what happens, basically. I did a couple of little rescues in the north corner of Maroubra, but that was about it. At Coogee you did nothing. You don't realise what the lifeguards do till you spend some time there. If Hoppo and Box aren't there I'm the team leader, so that can be stressful at times. But we do all we can, that's the duty of care covered.'

There are many things a lifeguard sees that no amount of training will anticipate. The other day Deano came across a bloke down at the water's edge with a bottle of olive oil, baptising himself. When Dean gently suggested he move on, the baptisee began muttering, 'Leave me alone, I just wanna be alone.' There were about 20,000 people on the beach at the time. 'When there's no rescues going on, all this other stuff finds you ... it makes you wonder what happens when we're busy. People getting taken photos of, all that stuff. Rather be busy doing rescues.'

> Dean doesn't seem worried by the idea of a TV camera. 'I sorta pretend they're not there ... just get on with the job.'

Then there's fun stuff, like the little Port Jackson shark in the north end babies' pool one morning. 'We got a broom and one of those black plastic recyclable bins and we were chasing it around the pool. Couldn't get it in. So eventually we broomed it into the shallow bit and I grabbed it by the tail. There was a crowd by then and they were all clapping ... I thought, "How cool's this shit? I'm an adrenaline junkie and this is my WORK! How good's this!"'

If Dean's been worried at times by the one truly unusual aspect of his job—the fact that he's regularly watched doing it by a considerable TV audience—he's learned to put that in perspective too. 'I sorta pretend they're not there,' he says of the cameras. 'Just get on with the job. I think that works.'

Besides, the show has changed a few minds in his own family circle. 'It's funny, Mum's a nurse and she'd have seen some amazing stuff at work, and one of my friends is a copper, and they just say, "I can't believe what you do at work!" And I say "I told ya so" a thousand times, and they say "Yeah, but to see it firsthand ..."'

His dad used to try to persuade Dean to 'get a real job', but no longer. Indeed, beyond lifeguarding as well as in it, Dean's doing OK. He does personal training for a small list of clients; the evidence, in the shape of fit balls and other gear, is strewn around the apartment.

Meanwhile he's engaging with an intriguing turn of family events. At 54, Dean's dad has just had a baby daughter with his new partner. Now Dean is due to be the best man at his dad's second wedding, a prospect that sounds as if it's thrown him ever so slightly.

'I paid $20 to look at a website called "Best man's speeches", and it says some people are cut out for making speeches and others just aren't!' He laughs. 'I think that's me. Just as long as I don't try to talk too much. Tell a few jokes and leave it there.'

wild stories FROM THE SERVICE

The Ring of Death

ON KUTA BEACH, June 2008. Harries is sunbaking and trying to make friends with the girls, kidding them he's Chief Lifeguard. Deano's not far away. They look south down the beach—Kuta is long and flat and open in both directions—and see a crowd gathered in one spot.

At first they think it's a volleyball game; then they realise it's a gathering of an entirely different kind, the kind the lifeguards call a Ring of Death—people gathered in a circle around one person or persons washed or carried from the surf.

The pair take off at a dead run towards the ring, 3 kilometres away, what looks like around 200 people clustered around a man and a woman. There's an American doctor already on the spot, asking for oxygen and trying to walk the man around despite the fact that he's unconscious and not breathing. Harries and Deano crash the circle and immediately begin EAR—expired-air resuscitation, the technique used when no oxygen-delivery system is available—and get a grip on the situation. Then a bemo-style ambulance arrives, roaring down the sand, dogs and dust in its wake. The rear doors fly open and the attendants lift up the girl—who's the worst off—and slide her into the back, where Deano and Kris Yates get to work with the oxygen. Harries feels a moment of relief, which instantly ends when the attendants slam the bemo's doors shut and roar off back up the sand, leaving him with the Ring of Death and a dying man under his hand. 'It's an amazing feeling,' he says, 'having someone dying in your arms.' Astonishingly, after a dash through the Kuta back streets on the back of the Bali guards' recently acquired ATV, the man survives.

Struck by lightning

THE END OF a busy day, a big thunderstorm builds quickly with an approaching southerly. The beach soon clears as people take off, avoiding the rain on the horizon, and the guards are laughing, thinking it's going to be an easy finish to the day. Hurray for the thunderstorm! Then ... BOOM! Dr Colin O'Brien, out from Ireland and at the beach with some friends, is struck down by a bolt from the storm, and flat-lines on the spot. Deano is one of those on duty. 'I see the boys running down the beach,' he says. 'We got him on the bike and brought him up and started resuscitating. His friends were yelling at us and we were yelling at them, until they could see we knew what we were doing. Then we started rotating CPR on him. It took about fifteen minutes. Some ambos turned up and we kept going. They attached a defib. We got a pulse, lost a pulse, and kept going till we got it again.' Almost incredibly, the patient survives; six months later, still in recovery and confined to a wheelchair, he pays the lifeguards a visit to say thanks. Deano says, 'Colin! I can still remember them calling his name—"Come on Colin! Come on Colin!"'

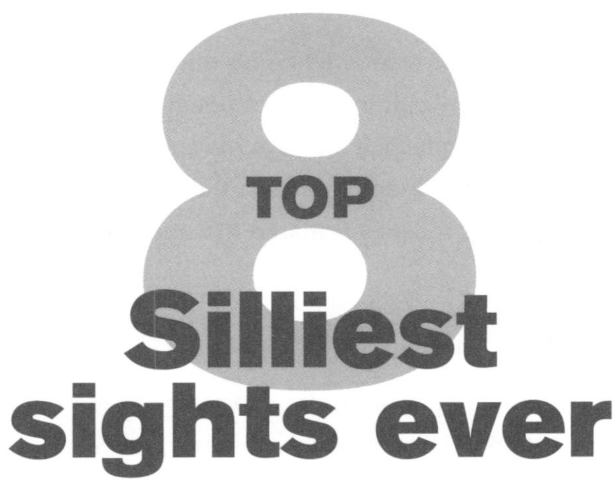

TOP 8 Silliest sights ever

Along with all the people who can't swim charging into the water, and the people who walk to the tower carrying a bluebottle and wondering why it hurts, some things just stand out:

1. The kite-surfer

The sport's not permitted at Bondi, for good reason–the kite strings can be dangerous as hell in even a minor crowd. One man decided to go anyway, and when the boys called him in, the wind did the rest, pulling surfer and kite across the sand and bang into the promenade. The footage made it into Bondi legend.

2. Wombat exercise

At first Harries thought it was a dog–just a very stumpy dog. But when he got down on the sand to ask the 'dog's' owner to move his pet off the beach, he found it was in fact a wombat. The Bondi Wombat! Harries now knows the correct way to lift a wombat, by the way, so if you're ever in need …

3. The ski beaching

Whippet owns a jet ski with a few other surfers for towing-in on big days, so when the service was down a ski, he happily loaned it. He didn't count on lifeguard Kris Yates 'beaching' it with such vigour that it crash-tackled one of the ATVs. Yatesy's still living it down. 'Broke a brand-new rescue board,' reports Ryan. 'Nothing wrong with the ski though.'

4. Paris Hilton crowds

The celebrity heiress never fails to enliven her fellow visitors to Bondi. 'People trail round behind her,' says Deano, 'it's like a human comet! They'll do anything to get a glimpse, it's pathetic but hilarious too.'

5. Board meets boat

It's a nice day in the southern corner, a surf club inshore rescue boat crew is on a training run ... they're on their way out just as a novice surfer on a longboard picks up a wave ... neither party corrects course in time ... CRASH! ... and the surfer does a backflip off his board ... and lands directly in the IRB. 'Couldn't have planned it,' reckons Kerrbox.

6. The exploding man

A temporary resident of the southern rocks was busy with a bottle of methylated spirits. 'He said he was practising fire-twirling,' says Dean, 'but he was drinking it–obviously.' Anyway, this candidate for the Darwin Awards lit a cigarette and blew himself up; came running down the rocks in a panic, fell over and broke his leg.

7. The horse is loose

A crowded summer day and a policeman on horseback; a pretty enough picture until the horse, for whatever reason, panics, throws its human cargo, and takes off. The horse proceeds to gallop the length of the beach, with cop in hot pursuit. 'You felt sorry for the guy,' says Tom, 'but you had to laugh.'

8. Up, up and away

This one goes out to the guy who recently set himself up in a chair on the promenade with two dozen helium-filled balloons attached, planning to lift off the ground, for a dare. 'I'll pop 'em one by one to come back down,' he told Harries. Never got up–thank Huey.

BILL MORRIS

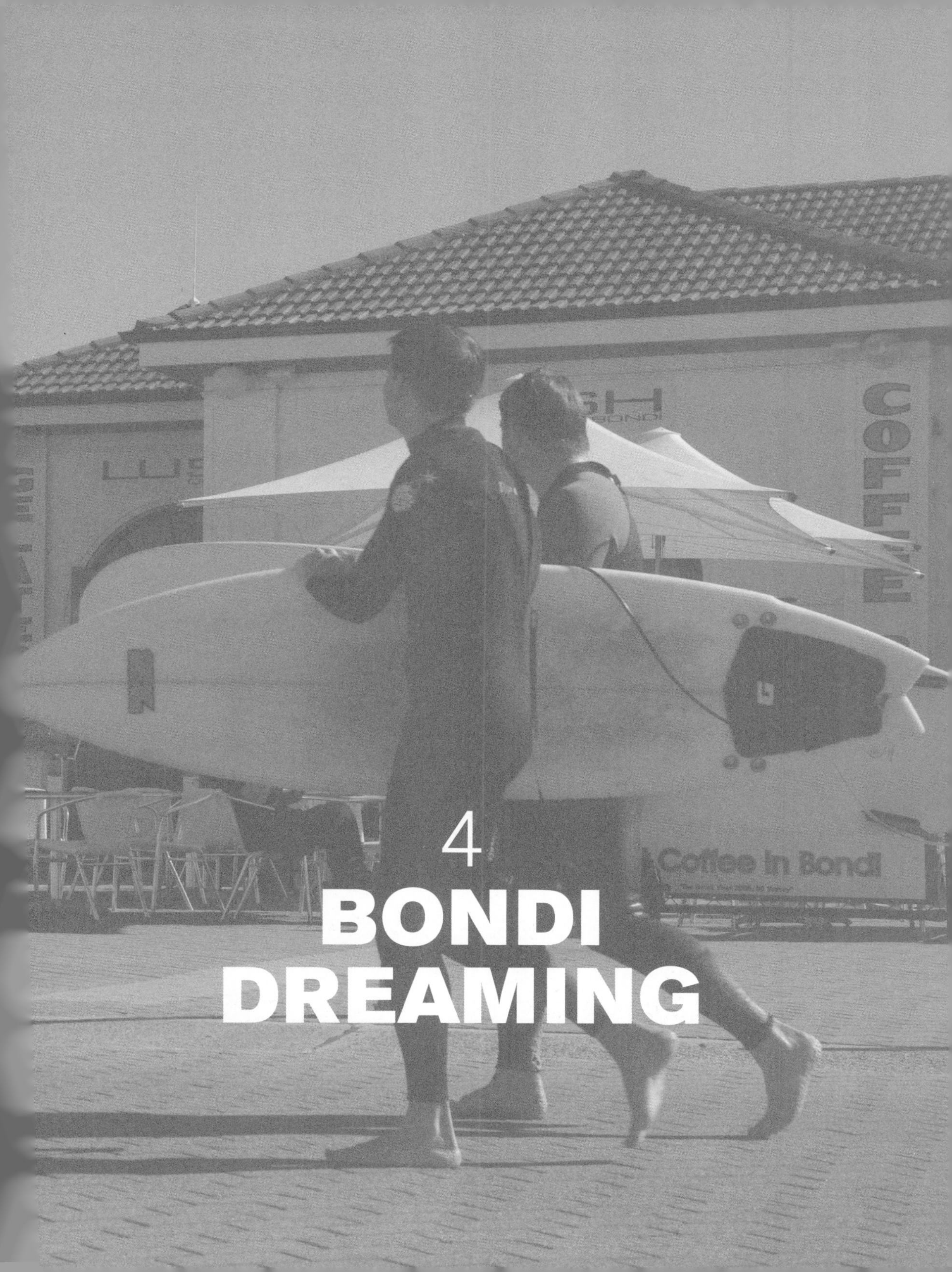

4
BONDI DREAMING

How does a kilometre of white-sand beach become iconic?

It's 900 metres along the high-tide line, a kilometre along the promenade. In between, like the teeth in a model's smile, is the curved stretch of white gleaming sand we know as Bondi Beach. Star of the show.

Standing high on the southern hill on a January morning among the stunted pandanus and Norfolk pines, you can watch the migrations towards that gleaming sand: hungover kids from the backpacker hostels carrying their surfboards-for-hire, glossy young women on pre-lunch power walks, men in sunglasses and tight-buttoned shirts exiting Mercedes on Notts Avenue, uni students on half-day breaks, hapless inhabitants of tour buses, skateboarders, junkies. 'It's the Kings Cross of the beaches,' says Tom Bunting. 'When I think of Australian culture, I think of the bush and I think of the beach, and I guess when people hear the word "Bondi" they think of the beach. When people come down here in summer it turns into one big party. It's chaos.'

The lifeguards have a complex set of reactions to their glamorous workplace. They're at once over-familiar and quite clear-eyed. Perhaps they've seen too much of it. Hoppo, for example, thinks Bondi is a bit overrated: 'If you look around Australia there's a lot of beaches that look a lot better. I don't know why it's become such an icon.'

Perhaps the answer is partly in its urban surrounds. Bondi is indeed an Australian icon, yet it's the most European of Aussie beaches: framed by walls, promenade, pavilions, hotels, and rows and rows of tightly packed flats and houses, it's anything but a typical east coast beach. Even the direction it faces, south-east, is off-line with most of its Sydney cousins. But this provides the beach's strength—protection from the summer north-easterly sea breeze, which fans Bondi from the side rather than striking it head-on, highlighting that magical water colour. The white sand reflects sun-light almost like snow, turning the whole remarkably broad beach into a solar tanning salon.

The beach's angle is also its greatest danger to unwary swimmers, exposing them to occasional shock visits from far-off Southern Ocean storms—deep, hidden groundswells that arrive without warning or connection with local weather. Just such a set of waves arrived at Bondi about 80 years ago on 6 February 1938, around 3 p.m. Three waves were in the set, not huge, but thick in the manner of a long groundswell, and they hit in perfect succession, spaced just far enough apart that the impact of each was maximised. The next hour has been inscribed in Bondi legend as 'Black Sunday', as surf lifesavers, hindered by panicky crowds, dragged around 250 people out of the water. Four died there on the white sands.

The word 'bondi' is variously claimed to mean 'noise of water breaking over rocks' or 'flight of the nullas' (a 'nulla' is a club or throwing stick used in battle). Prior to European settlement, the nearest Aboriginal mob was the Birrabirragal, who spoke the Sydney dialect Dharug, but spent most of their time in the harbourside of the peninsula, around what's known now as Watson's Bay. The

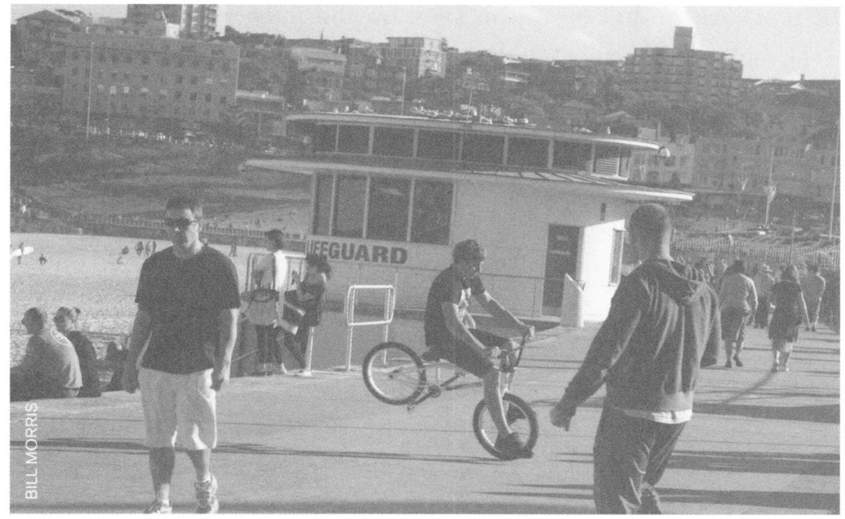

ABOVE The promenade lends Bondi an almost European vibe.

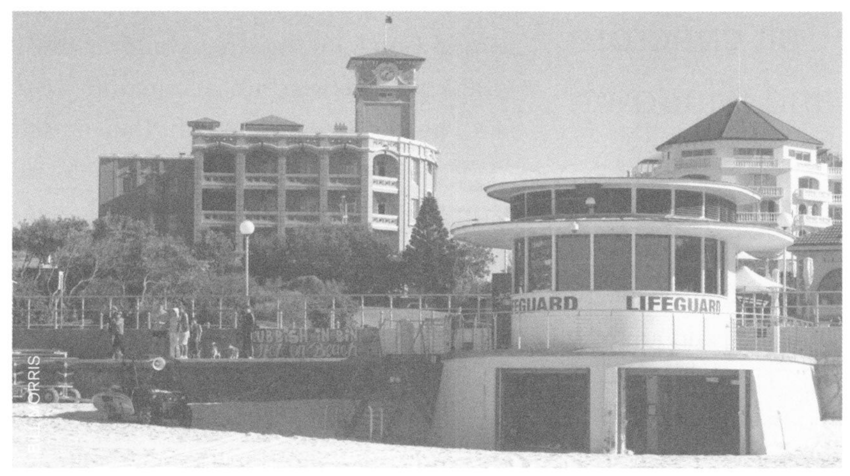

ABOVE Beneath the tower runs the old access tunnel, dating back to the 1920s.

Birrabirragal didn't seem too keen on the noise of water breaking over rocks. Neither for some time were the European settlers. In the 1850s, when the local landowner Francis O'Brien first threw it open to picnickers, the Bondi coast was still largely untouched, with big sandhills rising up to the north-west ridge.

The lifeguard tower is the boys' little castle on the sand: an odd little circular space, all concrete and windows.

Francis's attempts to subdivide the sandhills weren't greeted with much enthusiasm. But the appearance of a dance hall and a pub evoked more than mere enthusiasm. On Boxing Day 1884, Bondi delivered a taste of the busy days to come; the first hint of Tom's 'chaos'. 'The pretty little village was crowded with visitors,' reported the *Sydney Morning Herald*, 'and amongst them were some members of the larrikin type.' Oh, those larrikins! They attended the Cliff House Hotel, on the site of today's Astra, drank themselves into a splendid state, and headed for the Bondi Dance Hall right next door. The results: a colossal and spectacular all-in brawl, three policemen chased into the bushes and beaten up, three rioters sentenced to several years' jail, and the cancellation of the Bondi Dance Hall's licence, on the grounds of 'nuisance and annoyance to the inhabitants'.

The infamous riot of 1884 would be tale enough without the fact that exactly 110 years later, on Boxing Day 1994, the whole scene was more or less repeated. This time the rioters were mostly young—backpacker-style tourists and visitors from other parts of Sydney who'd decided the hill between Bondi's main drag, Campbell Parade, and the pavilion was the right place to get really drunk. Again some cops were hurt, again some arrests were made. But now Bondi wasn't just sandhills and a dance hall; it was expensive real estate and glitzy stores and restaurants, and it had a council willing to ban drinking on the beach.

These days the closest anyone gets to rioting is when Paris Hilton performs a stage-walk along the sands. Larrikinism may be part of Bondi, but it's taken a back seat to starpower—for now.

In 1928, the enclosing promenade was completed, along with a couple of long concrete tunnels reaching out across the beach, almost to the water's edge. Down these tunnels would pour the beach-going hordes, fed from changing sheds set up within the pavilion. During World War II, the tunnels were dynamited for fear of Japanese invasion, but the parts beneath the promenade remain intact.

Above the remnant of the southern tunnel, which is stacked with rescue boards and other gear, is the lifeguard tower: the boys' little castle on the sand. It's an odd little circular space, all concrete and windows. There's a CCTV screen drawing off a camera mounted on the front, controlled by a joystick; it can be zeroed in on any point on the beach, but the lifeguards rely more on the binoculars. There's an old Waverley Municipal Council (WMC) life ring, a blown-up map of the Bondi coast and streets from a UBD directory, and a small pink David Hasselhoff clock hanging above the window frame. There's a tiny fridge full of Red Bull. And way up on one of the upper window frames, there's a cut-out circle of paper with a deformed caricature of Box drawn on it.

'High enough so he can't reach it,' reckons Dean.

Harries points out the differences between Bondi and its less crowded yet more turbulent neighbour beaches. Bronte's very family oriented: mostly locals, some people from elsewhere, but by and large the haunt of swimmers and surfers familiar with the ocean's moods. They have to be. Bronte's size and shape tends to magnify any kind of surf, and it's flanked with lots of cliff line, meaning rescues there are usually full-on—but there are way less of them. At Bondi, he says, 'You become a lot like a ferry service. You're pulling in a lot more tourists there, dealing with a lot more dramatic situations, like 100 bluebottle stings at once, or a guy who'll walk up to the tower and say, "Listen I'm not feeling the best", and die in your arms.'

Celebrities, wannabe drug dealers, steroid heads, according to Harries: 'They all seem to fit into their own little slot down there. It's the Hollywood of the coast.'

The lifeguards have their own social geography, their own map, dividing the beach up between its tribes: 'We get the gays and families at North Bondi, all the kids and tourists in the main section, then all the backpackers from second or third ramp down to the south corner, mainly because that's where the backpacker hostels are,' says Kerrbox. 'The backpackers don't come down till 3 p.m. The families are usually gone by lunch and the kids in the middle are going mad all day.'

Like the other guards, Tom points out the multiplicity of cultures, but his interests are different: 'I got this great recipe off this Indian family who were down at the beach; they had some of this naan bread and they were more than happy to swing me a couple of slices. I ended up with the recipe and it's great. Just one of the little perks of the job.' (It's a different idea of 'perk' than, say, Harries's might be.)

Corey Oliver, on the other hand, notes the weird shit, the thieves, the freaks: 'Bondi's such an iconic place to the world but there's still this little dark space, it's really high end and low end.

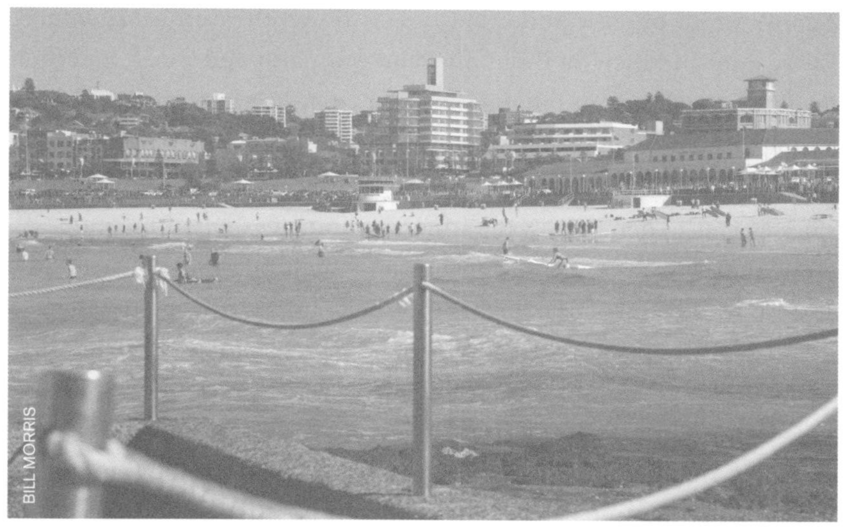

ABOVE Endlessly defined by water.
Bondi from the Icebergs pool.

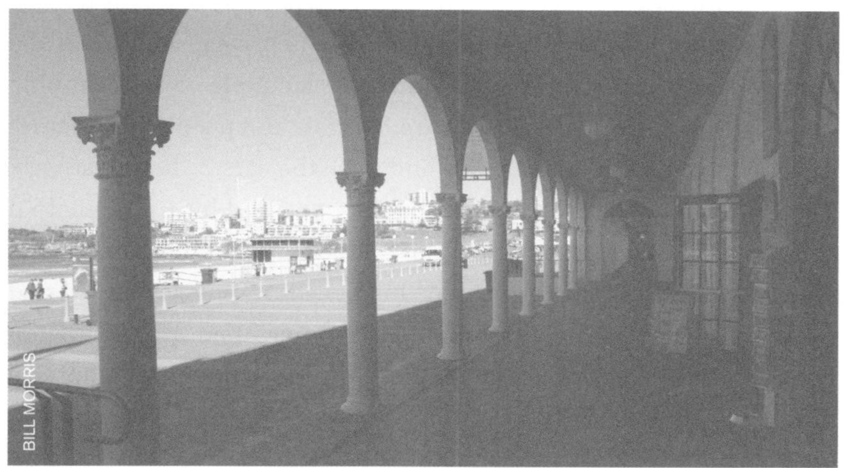

ABOVE The Pavilion's pillar frame
strikes a wacky classical touch.

There's quite often a dude that comes down dressed as a woman. Every now and then he'll put on some war paint and a veil, and high heels, and walk around in the sand. He's a messed-up unit. He's a big strong guy and you're not sure whether to ask him to leave or not. He'll walk along doing his thing, and then stop and peg you out, stare at you.' Then there's the itinerant homeless, often mentally ill, who wallow around in the bushes and such behind the surf clubs and pavilion. A lot of beaches are like that—home to fringe-dwellers—but this one seems to draw more than its share, again perhaps because of the urbanity, the opportunity of a free feed or a dropped wallet.

Corey reminds his visitor of the old bloke living in the south end cliff. He's been there seven years—a flashback to the Depression years, when humpies full of unemployed families dotted the South Bondi headland. Corey points out a simple fact of life for that old bloke, the same reason others spend millions on apartments along Campbell Avenue: 'It's a good view.'

The forecast helps tell the lifeguards what sort of day it'll be. A surprise warm day won't necessarily mean carnage. But when the TV news weather forecast tells Sydney for a couple of days running that it's going to be 35 degrees on Wednesday, and people from across the city have time to make plans and pack the cars ... that's carnage. The guards will get up on a morning like that and by 1 p.m. there'll be thirty or forty thousand people scattered up and down. Deano is sure the numbers have increased this decade: 'When I first started people would come to the beach in summer, then around March nobody would come down any more. Nowadays if you get a hot day in September, there'll be about 35,000 people down the beach. And only a couple of lifeguards doing winter staff. Mayhem!'

The widely travelled Box compares it to Rio de Janeiro in Brazil for crowd size; maybe also Huntington Beach in California. But those spots are wide open, whereas Bondi is enclosed by its headlands, the chaos concentrated. Between 3 p.m. and 5 p.m., they'll have sharks, a bashing, helicopters, a spinal injury, all at the same time. Deano says, 'Any major incident will take two lifeguards out of the game; you can only afford to have so many things at once, yet they so often do seem to happen together.'

Yet beyond all the chaos and humanity and urbanity, there's still that model-smile arc of sand, and the water beyond. The biggest change along Sydney's coast in the past 20 years has been the relocation of the sewage outfall system. Today most of Sydney's treated sewage is released several kilometres to sea in deep water, and never comes back to the coastline. But prior to that, the sewage was released directly into coastal waters through a series of cliff-face outfalls. One of the biggest was at North Bondi. The result? 'There was this huge plume of shit going out off the headland,' says Kerrbox. 'North Bondi was a sewer outlet. It was disgusting. Every time a nor-easter blew in you could smell the shit. You'd feel sick, it was horrible, this big brown stain.'

Today, it's gloriously different. Each year the memory of the sewage days falls further away; the sea seems to glow with rude blue health, and schools of kingfish and Australian salmon come in to the bay. The potential downside, shark presence, has a passing impact, yet people still seem keener than ever on the Australian icon. Says Kerrbox, 'It's the best I've seen it.'

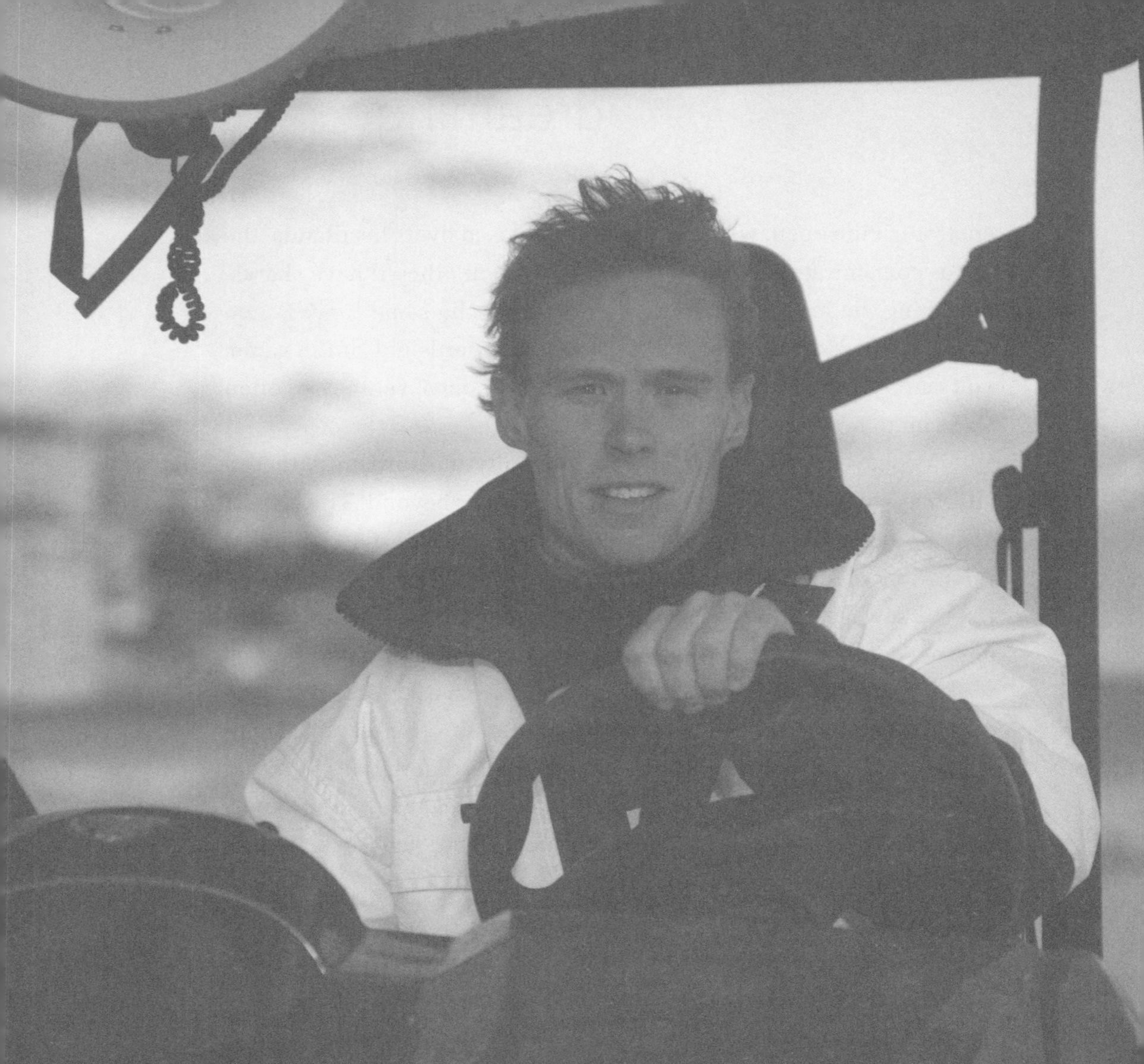

BILL MORRIS

Reidy: The Live Wire
(Andrew Reid)

It's hard to be sure of anything at Bondi, but one thing is almost guaranteed: Within moments of meeting him, Andrew Reid will be asking you questions. 'Do you know any good books on photography?' he says, betraying his recent fascination with the lens. 'Have you looked at frothers.com?' he asks, naming the local surf website run by one of the lifeguards. 'I've got a couple of shots on there.'

Reidy has a quick mind, questioning and eager for information, so he talks fast, energetically, in a very traditional Aussie accent. When he smiles or squints against the sun, both of which happen often, his eyes form triangular slits, the skin wrinkling down from above and below, pushing up from prominent cheekbones. It's an old style of Australian face, one you might see on a cricketer or a jockey, an effect accentuated by his slim frame and quick physical movements. Reidy can stay still about as long as a sparrow.

Right now he's sitting at an outside table at one of south Bondi's many cafes, eating an ultra-healthy fruit plate for lunch and waving away anyone's attempts to pay. 'You're a guest in my town,' he says.

'Hey—I wanted to ask—do you know any good sports biographies? I wanna get psyched up for the Lifeguard Challenge!'

It's almost impossible to square up this current version of Andrew Brian Reid against the person he describes at the age of fourteen—fat, unmotivated, struggling at school, and about as interested in the beach as, say, Marilyn Manson. But maybe that's Reidy. The only kid in the lifeguard tower without an intensive surfing background, he wouldn't be sitting here talking about critical resuscitations and how to deal with huge beach crowds if he wasn't able to reinvent himself at need … and if he wasn't fundamentally a ball of energy.

Reidy was born on 3 June 1979, in Paddington Women's Hospital, has an older and a younger sister, and three much older half-brothers from his dad's previous marriage.

Mum, Trish, was daughter of a navy man—Rear-Admiral Thomas Kenneth Morrison—and she travelled a lot, did a bit of nursing. Reidy can't remember Rear-Admiral Morrison, but he's heard many stories and seen the pictures with the Queen. The Admiral's daughter met Brian Reid around 30 years ago, after Brian's first wife had died. Brian grew up around Clovelly, and sounds as if he was keen on high speeds; according to his son, he was in a Mini-Minor club called the Crack-A-Ton Club. 'You had to break the 100 over a mile. There was a special corner down in Rose Bay that you had to … anyway he was a truck mechanic, a used-car salesman.'

Andrew grew up in Vaucluse, and though they were a swimming-oriented family—he joined the Nippers along with sisters Kirsty and Kate, and Kirsty went on to be a top swim racer at North Bondi SLSC, nearly making the Australian team for the Pan Pacific Games—he was never much of a beach kid. Instead, the family spent a lot of time up on the Hawkesbury River, satisfying Brian and Trish's stoke on

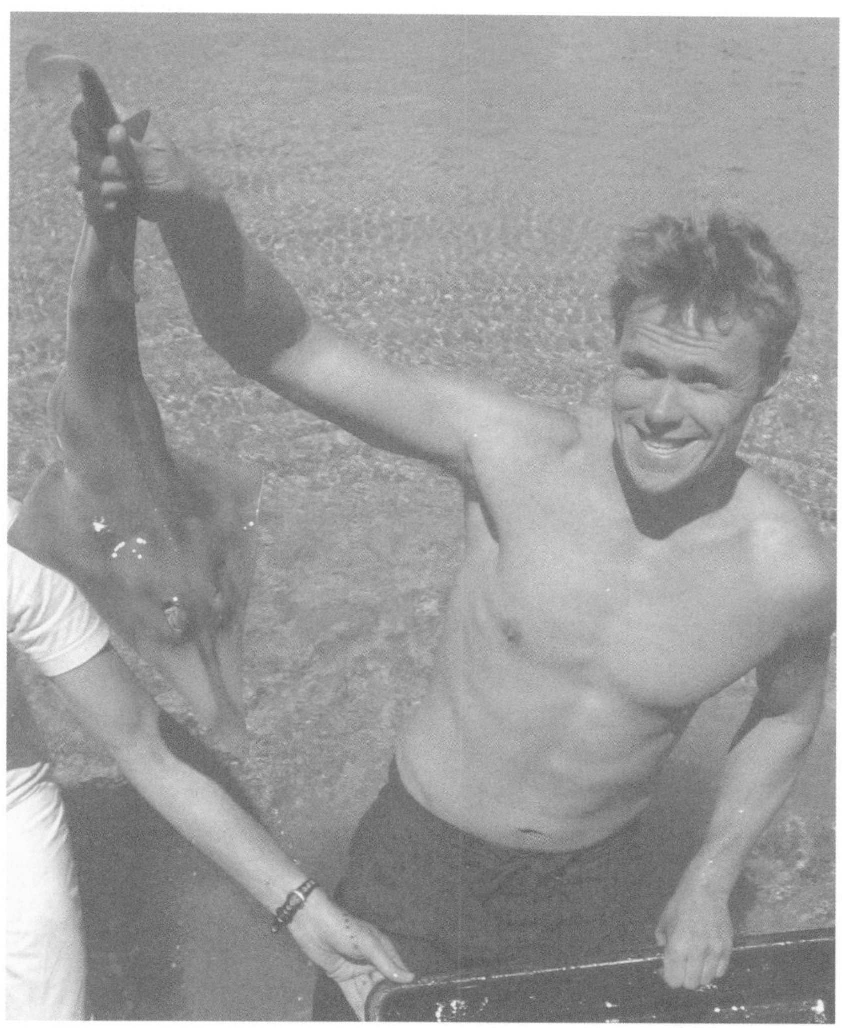

ABOVE Got to know your sea life.
Shovel-nose shark on a surf trip.

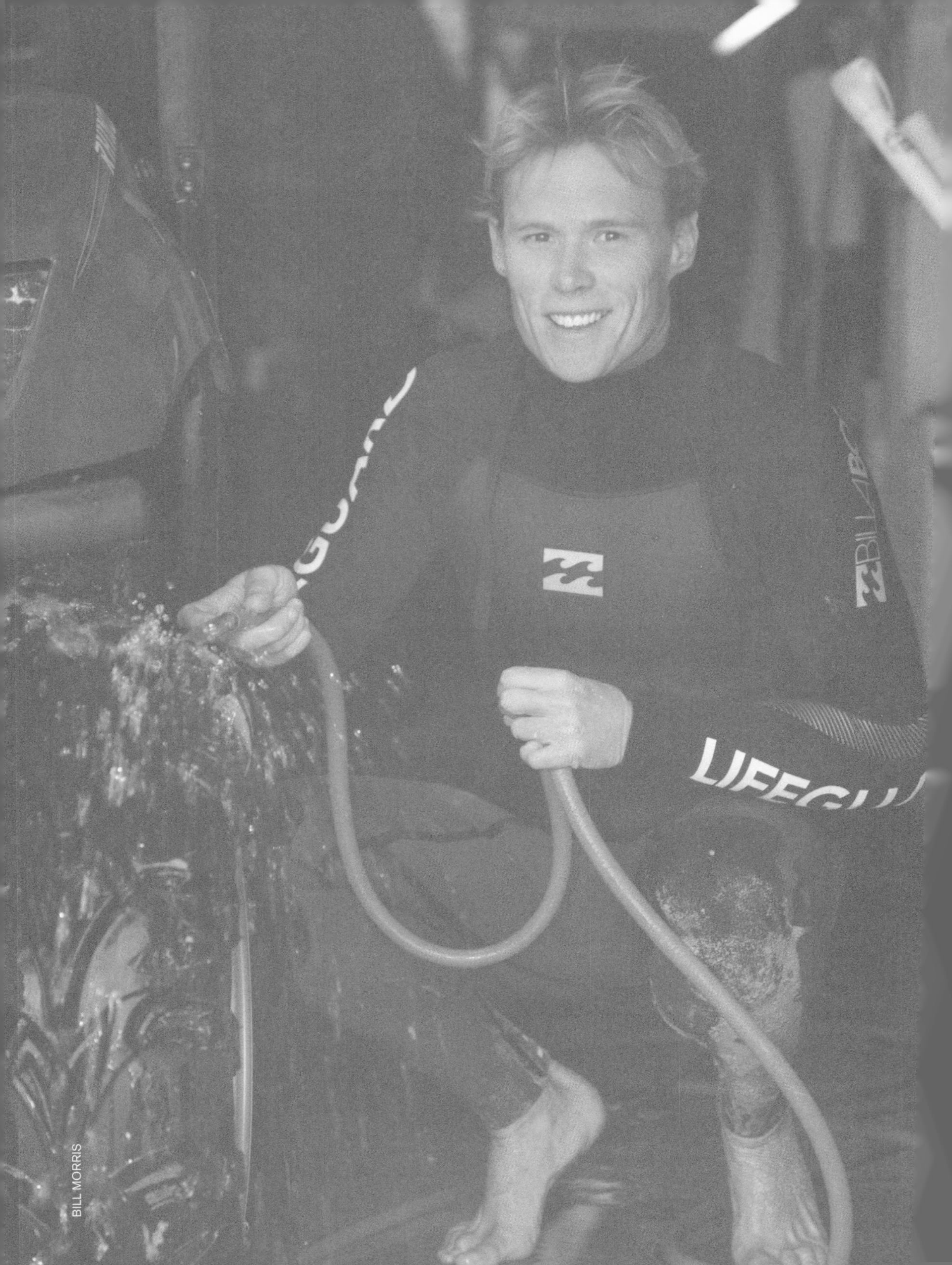

BILL MORRIS

waterskiing. Trish bought a 5-acre block on the river and built a nice house on it, and that was the destination on most weekends and holidays. Brian would rocket around behind their boat on one ski, balancing young Andrew on his shoulders. 'I had my friends at school, but apart from that we were away, so I didn't really hang out with anyone around here,' he says.

Reidy wasn't exactly un-sporty; he played tennis, and was coached professionally. His parents scraped up the money to send him to Waverley College, a nearby Catholic school. But something went wrong. Reidy didn't like Waverley College. He tells stories of avoiding school day after day, along with a mate whose mum gave them $50 to spend on junk food. He put on a lot of weight, and when he bothered to go to school, he hung out the back of the class with a similarly slack crew.

'My dad had big hopes for me but it just wasn't my thing,' he says. 'I got into pot, smoked a lot of pot. I was a bit of a rat. By Year 8, I wasn't getting into a lot of trouble but I wasn't going to school, I was smoking dope. Eventually Mum said, "OK, that's the end of that." She went out and got another job driving disabled kids to school, earned some money and sent me off to Bathurst, of all places, to a boarding school. I lasted a day there. They took us around the school and I just said, "I can't stay here." I ran away. Just ran into the cornfields. Mum said, "Right, you can go to Dover with your sisters." So I ended up at Dover.' Dover Heights High—Hoppo's old school—had a bad reputation at the time, but somehow Reidy fell in with a really good bunch of schoolmates. He was ridiculed for being

LEFT Reidy's never happier than when he's doing something. Anything! Washing off the rhino.

overweight, but he stopped smoking dope, got back into studying, got back into playing tennis, and things slowly turned around.

'When I was sixteen or so I had a crush on a girl,' he says. 'I was still really overweight. It was New Year's Eve and I tried to hook up with her, and she said no. She didn't tell me it was because I was fat, but I knew that was why … you could tell.' He devoted the next year to losing the weight, had a short slightly vengeful relationship with his former crush, and got on with life.

Some time after finishing school, Reidy went to the United States for a working holiday teaching waterskiing at a summer camp, a job that involved some lifeguarding. Back in Australia, he took a job as a Waverley Council garbage truck runner—a job he still does part-time and in the lifeguarding off-season—and realised he enjoyed the hard physical work. 'I thought I might try and get a bit fit. Went to the gym and got fitter and began going down to the beach again. Watched the lifeguards and thought, "Gee, that'd be a good job".' One of his fellow garbos, a surfer from Maroubra named Matt Phillips, was working as a lifeguard as well, and suggested he try out for the service. 'He threw a good word in with Hoppo, and I trained, and tried out and got in and the rest is history,' he laughs.

Reidy started at Bondi in 2002. Since then he's performed around 50 critical rescues, ones where the patient is either unconscious or in serious danger of drowning; four or five of them have been without a pulse. 'The typical rescue? I don't think there is one. They're all different and you don't know which one you'll get. You get the English backpackers, they scream and make lots of noise and fight for their life. Some of 'em you can hear 'em screaming from the tower. Then you've got the Asians who don't do a lot of screaming, but they do a shitload of thrashing. Some from the mid-European countries will use their wife's head as a stool to climb up on.

There's nothing general. It is mostly backpackers but there's nothing general about 'em.'

'Some people are lucky here because so much is going on, there's so many other people around, they'll get saved by some surfer, and we won't even hear about it.'

'The typical rescue? I don't think there is one. They're all different and you don't know which one you'll get.'

Reidy knew he didn't have the core surfing background of some of the others, and it caused him some stress at first. But Harry Nightingale has shown him a few things about Bondi that most people don't know: places to jump off, little holes that form and disappear. You get the sense that his willingness to ask questions served him well in this arena. 'When I first started doing this job I was shitting myself. But now I feel as soon as you know what's going on, you take a deep breath, remember what to do and go into that mode. And when you're working with the right guys, it's good. Nothing else matters apart from getting this person breathing. Everyone knows what to do and just goes into work.'

He lost a patient in the second series of the show, and it really cut him up, but his mum told him something that helped him deal with it—he hadn't got the person in that situation, it's not your fault, and you can only do your best.

The relationship with the surf clubs, does he think it works? 'Sometimes it does and sometimes it doesn't. They turn up on a Saturday or Sunday, ask us where we want 'em to put the tent, we tell 'em, then they put it right in front of where we don't want 'em to put it, and we have an argument about that. They drag patients into the tower, don't tell us about it and we have another argument about that. Other days—when we get along with 'em—fantastic! I think what the surf lifesaving movement does for the community is really good but you get the odd person down there who doesn't really wanna work in with us. They won't let us know about things when we have the responsibility.' Reidy did his Bronze for fun at Bronte surf club with his sister prior to being a lifeguard, so he has experience of both sides.

What he only half believes is that *Bondi Rescue* is making him famous. Reidy went to the Byron Bay Bluesfest after the first season and was stunned to realise that people could recognise him from the show. 'I'm just a garbo,' he mutters, screwing up his face in disbelief. 'Some people can't even believe I'm a garbo. I'm pulling their garbage bins out and they're looking at me like ... what?? They say, "But you're on a TV show!" I say, "Yeah, but I'm making really good money doing this".'

Today Reidy pictures himself as a future leader in the field; either that or he's got his eye on the ambulance service. 'I'm thinking about buying a place soon,' he says. His mum and dad still live in the same place where he grew up in Vaucluse, a small pretty house near Kincoppal School. Brian, the ex-member of the Crack-a-Ton Club, plays golf, and Trish does yoga five days a week. She's an early riser, as is Reidy, who's up at four most mornings. 'I'm only up at that hour because I'm a garbo,' he reckons.

Reidy is close to his sisters, but not to his half-brothers. One is a stonemason in Jindabyne. The other married a billionaire's daughter. Only one, Gary, the oldest, was around a bit when Reidy was a kid. Might see him now and then at Christmas.

In the 2009 season Reidy got closer to the show's production crew—thanks to Hoppo's scheduling trickery, he was employed on his off-days as a driver. Otherwise his season was a quiet one. 'I've done hardly any rescues. You could count 'em on two hands. I reckon it's because the show's working, to be honest … people stand up and take notice of us nowadays.'

The shark attack stands out in his mind as the single most dramatic event of the season, even though it happened outside lifeguard hours and the boys had left the beach half an hour before it occurred. 'I was at home and started getting a few phone calls from Kerrbox,' he recalls. 'I tend to ignore Kerrbox's phone calls after a certain time in the evening. But eventually I got a text from someone saying, "Shark attack! Unbelievable!"'

A little while later, Reidy the keen photographer took his water camera out on the back of a jet ski and dived on the shark nets for photos, just to see what he could find. 'Once you step off the ski sled, you're floating bait no matter what!' he says. 'I didn't see a hell of a lot, it was pretty murky down there. But I tell you what, when I came back up, I SPRINTED for that ski.'

wild stories FROM THE SERVICE

Reidy's flip

BY POPULAR ACCLAIM, Andrew Reid's the fastest rhino driver of the crew. One afternoon he's driving back up towards the tower, when Box spots a swimmer in trouble. 'Reidy! Go!' he yells over the radio. So Reidy hurls the rhino into a dramatic turn and takes off down the sand, full speed. What he seemingly hasn't noticed is the small berm—a ridge in the sand—that's formed as a result of heavy wave action. Reidy and the rhino explode over the edge of the berm ... The rescue board comes loose from its rack and spears into the lower sand layer ... The rhino pretty much stops dead and Reidy does a full somersault straight over the handlebars and, blam, onto the tarmac. Somehow he gets on with the job, albeit fairly groggily, while Kerrbox and the crew are in stitches in the tower. Once the rescue's completed, Reidy's getting his breath on the beach when a particularly attractive Brazilian girl strolls up and tells him, 'That's the funniest thing I've ever seen in my life.'

The pervert

THERE'S CONSIDERABLE PARANOIA in beach suburbs about the predatory photographer—the one who cruises the beach looking for chances to take photos of children in swimsuits. So one summer Sunday, when Hoppo gets a call about such a person prowling the north end—where a lot of families gather out of the wind and heavy surf—he heads off to investigate. Once there he spots actor Russell Crowe playing with his little son in a pool, looks up onto the road, and realises what's happening; up there in some bushes is the Sydney paparazzo Jamie Fawcett, trying to sneak off a few snaps of Crowe and kiddie at play. Then the whole thing goes ultra weird. 'We had the show's camera with us,' says Hoppo, 'and suddenly everyone thought WE were there to shoot Russell. They're all yelling, "Leave Russell alone, he's with his family", and this stuff. So we just pretended to stage an interview—as if the cameraman was interviewing me about something—but in fact he was shooting Russell the whole time over my shoulder. Basically, we became the paparazzi!' This job has endless hazards.

TOP 8 Bondi secrets

The beach is public property, yet it's a place with many private parts. Here are a few things that the lifeguards know ... and not many others do:

1. It's dangerous!

Bondi, the Aussie icon with its apparently calm blue waters, is in fact one of Sydney's riskier swimming beaches–especially for the 70-odd per cent of beach-goers who're non-swimming tourists. 'People drown here,' says Tom. Dean adds, 'It's just not something you'd automatically think of, but it's no piece of cake, even when it's small.'

2. Aboriginal art

There's a massive piece of Aboriginal art along the cliffs north of Bondi, facing seawards ... but you've got to be on the water in order to see it.

3. Shark Alley

The water trail along the northern cliff line out towards Ben Buckler was once known as 'Shark Alley', thanks to the large tiger sharks regularly caught by fishermen off the old boat ramp in pre-war times. Luckily they're not still at it today! However ...

4. Amazing marine life

Bondi boasts amazingly diverse marine life. The rocks are crusty with shellfish, and the bay is often full of schooling Australian salmon, tailor and other surface-feeding fish; whiting slither up and down the sandbar edges. 'You wouldn't expect it, this being a city beach and all that,' says Kerrbox, 'but it's incredibly clean.'

5. South–North is quickest

When swimming across the bay, it's quicker going from south to north than vice versa. This is because Bondi operates a bit like a big washing machine; water from broken waves pushes north to south along the shoreline, and recycles through the southern channel and Backpacker's Rip, heading out to sea and back to the quiet northern end.

6. Icebergs

If you're not up for that marathon, you can swim at Icebergs for a mere $3.

7. Sex on the beach

People have sex on the beach. A LOT. Especially on Sunday mornings when they think nobody's watching. 'Mostly backpackers,' reckons Harries.

8. Mornings

Australia's busiest and most urbanised beach is almost always beautiful and very peaceful early in the morning. 'You could be anywhere,' says Dean.

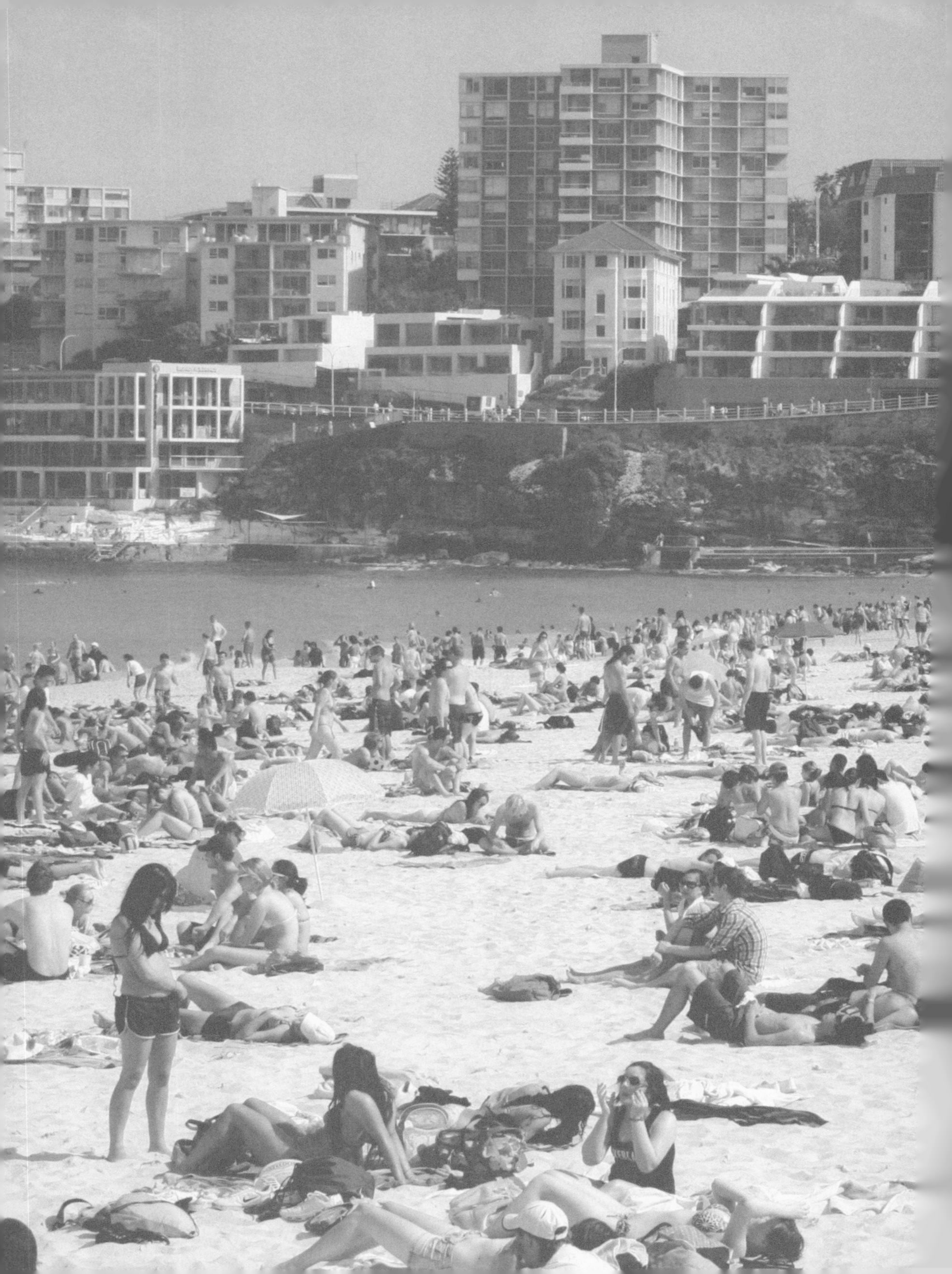

5 THE LONGEST DAY

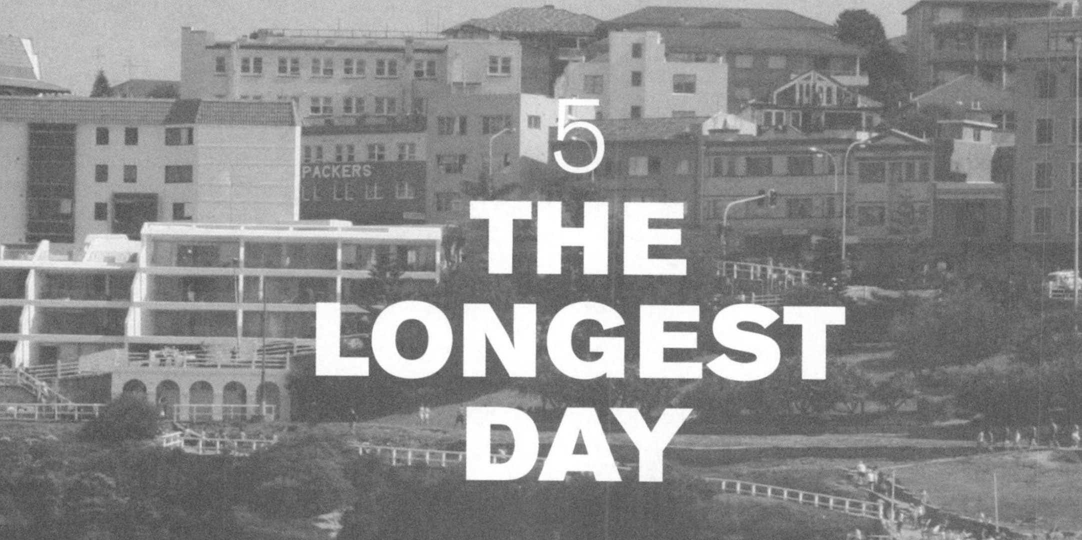

When things go wrong at Bondi, they really go wrong

Who hasn't heard of Black Sunday? It's the one day in Bondi Beach's long and wacky history that's pretty much impossible to avoid: 6 February 1938, the biggest mass rescue ever dealt with by surf clubs. That day, it's said, 250 people were rescued from the mess that three simple, thick, surprise waves had made of Bondi's central sandbar, and four died in the process.

It's become part of surf lifesaving's lore and legend, perhaps the central event in the SLSA's century-long existence.

Yet you've never heard of the Longest Day—a Friday afternoon in January 2005 when Bondi's on-duty lifeguard crew may well have exceeded Black Sunday's rescue figure. The official record filed with council says 235 rescues, but every lifeguard involved in that deceptively gentle day swears there were more—maybe many more. And all without losing a single life.

It happened in the midst of the wildest season in modern Bondi history—numerous near-drownings, resuscitations, retrievals, and all before the show was up and running. Why was 2004–05 such a big year for rescues? Perhaps it was a kind of critical mass moment, just before the series began its education of a new generation of beach-goers. Perhaps it was simply the beach itself. 'The rips were terrible all that summer,' Whippet says. 'I think we must have got a few swells in a row from different directions ... When there's a small swell from one angle for a couple of weeks, it just smooths everything out and flattens the sandbars. But if you get some north-east swell, then some south, then north-east again, the sand will get broken up and rips will form.'

Harries and his twin brother Sean were both on duty, along with Kerrbox and Andrew Reid. Reidy used to think you could predict a crazy Bondi day—that it had to be a Sunday, hot and sunny, enough to lure huge crowds from Sydney's immediate west. But the Longest Day was overcast, with a light onshore wind from the south-east, hardly dream summer weather. Nevertheless Harries recalls the rescue tally from the day prior as having been around 90. He says, 'The next morning I told Box, "Look there's gonna be 150 rescues today", and he said, "You're off your head".'

> 'We literally had bodies lying all over the beach ... there were 40,000 people on the beach and we just couldn't keep 'em out.'

Box confirms this. 'Well I opened my mouth that morning and said, "Boys it's sweet today, nothing's gonna happen, it's overcast and small, nice 'n easy today." At nine o'clock that night they were all, "You BASTARD! What were ya thinking?"'

Whippet's broken-up beach line set the scene. The surf was about 2 feet, only small, and there were two sandbanks shallow enough to stand on, but they were formed by rip action into horseshoe-like curves. When a little set of waves would

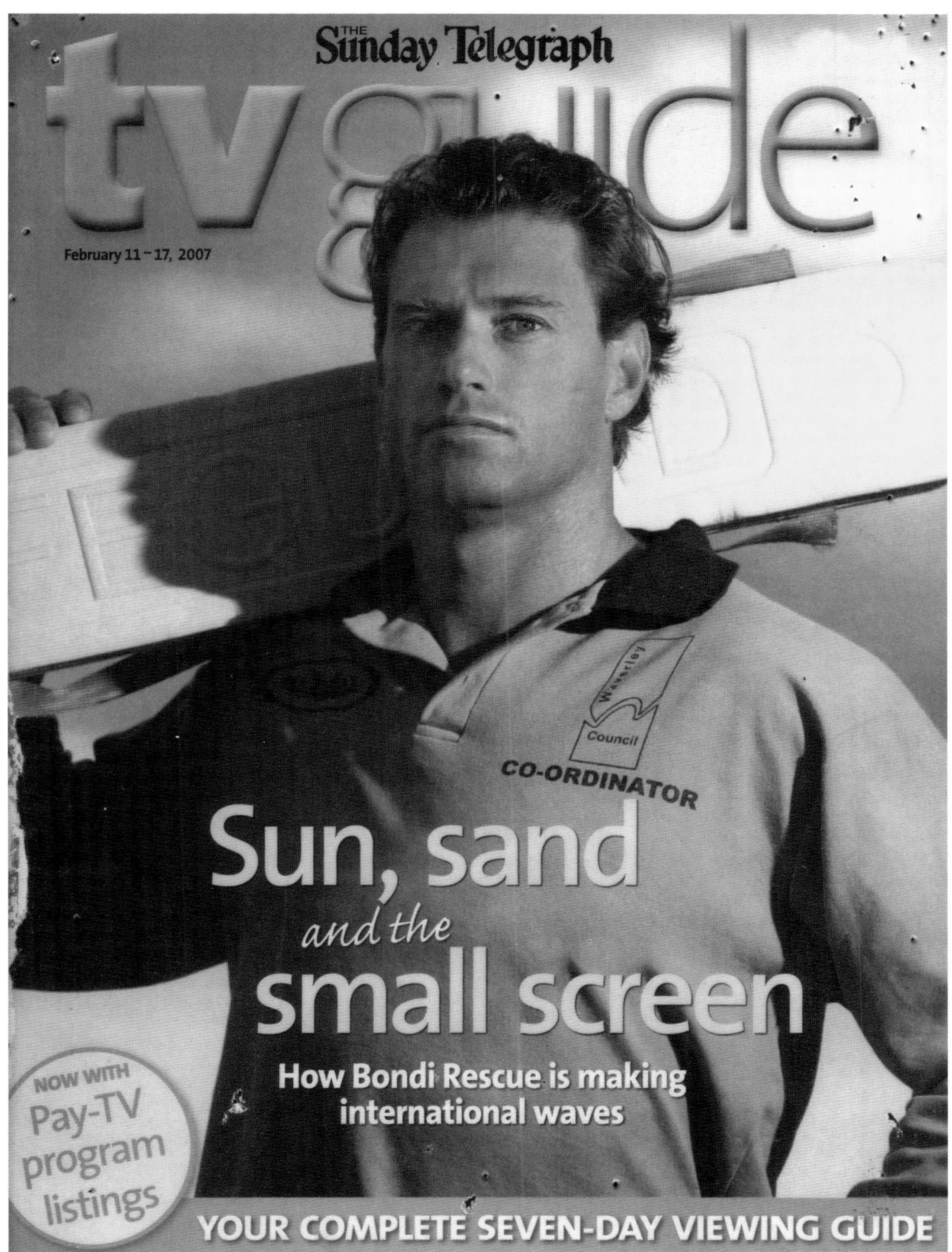

ABOVE Hoppo and the emblematic image that appeared on the *Sunday Telegraph*'s *TV Guide* cover: 'Sun, sand and the small screen.'

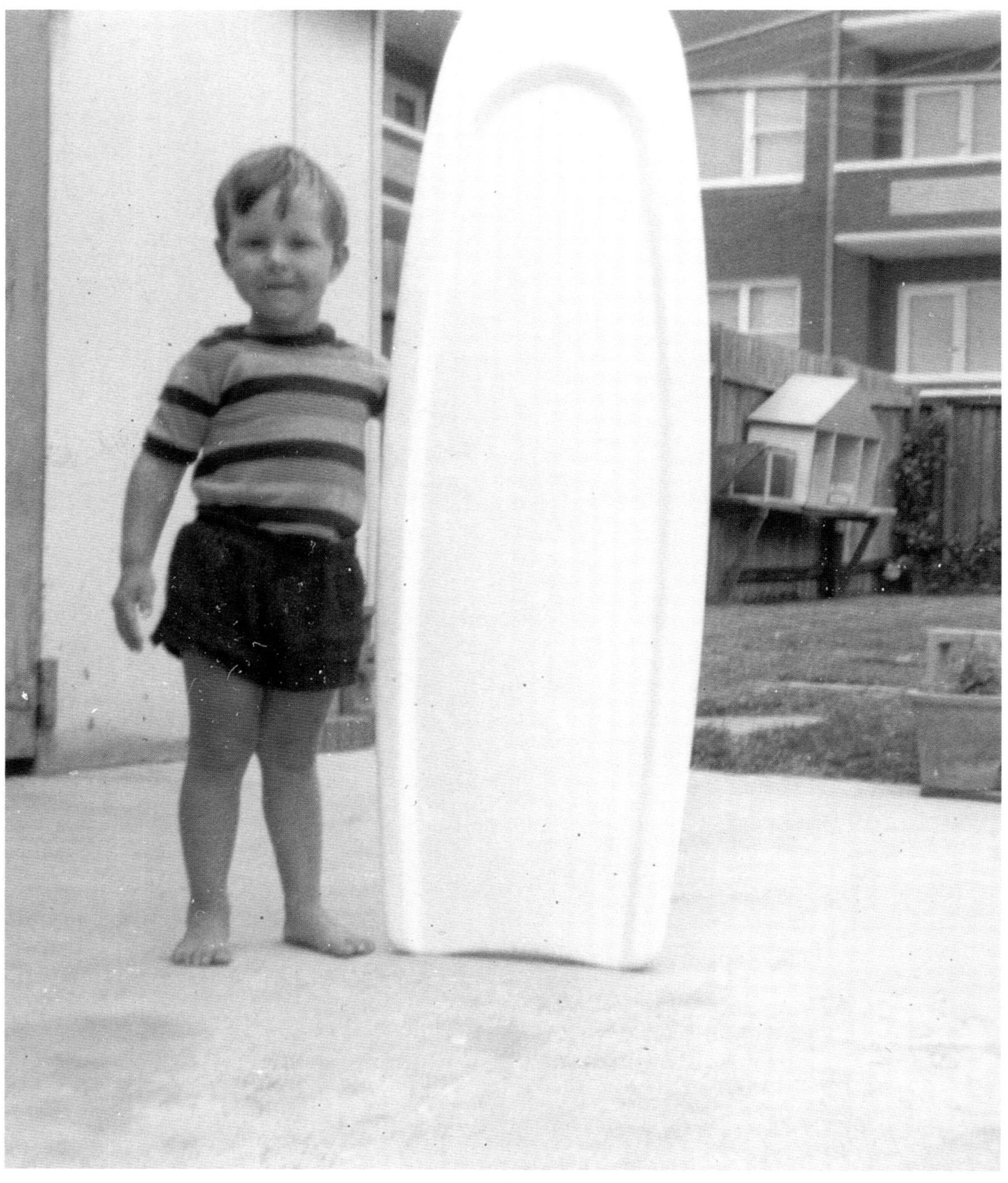

ABOVE Barely walking and he's already a larrikin. Rod 'Kerrbox' Kerr in the family backyard with every Aussie beach grommet's dream—his first Coolite surfboard.

TOP RIGHT Competition keeps you sharp. Hoppo and double ski teammate Tom Woodruff at a national carnival.

RIGHT 'Hi! I'm a TV star!' Yes Rodney, sure you are. Box on the tower with one of the show's Logies.

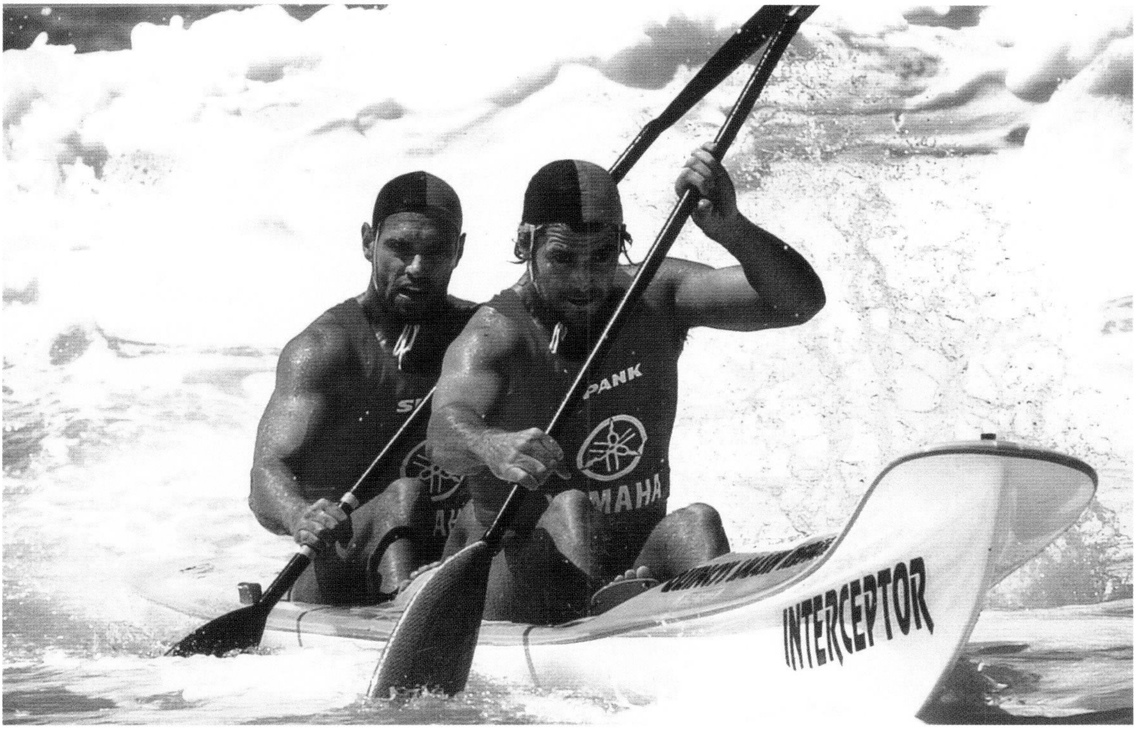

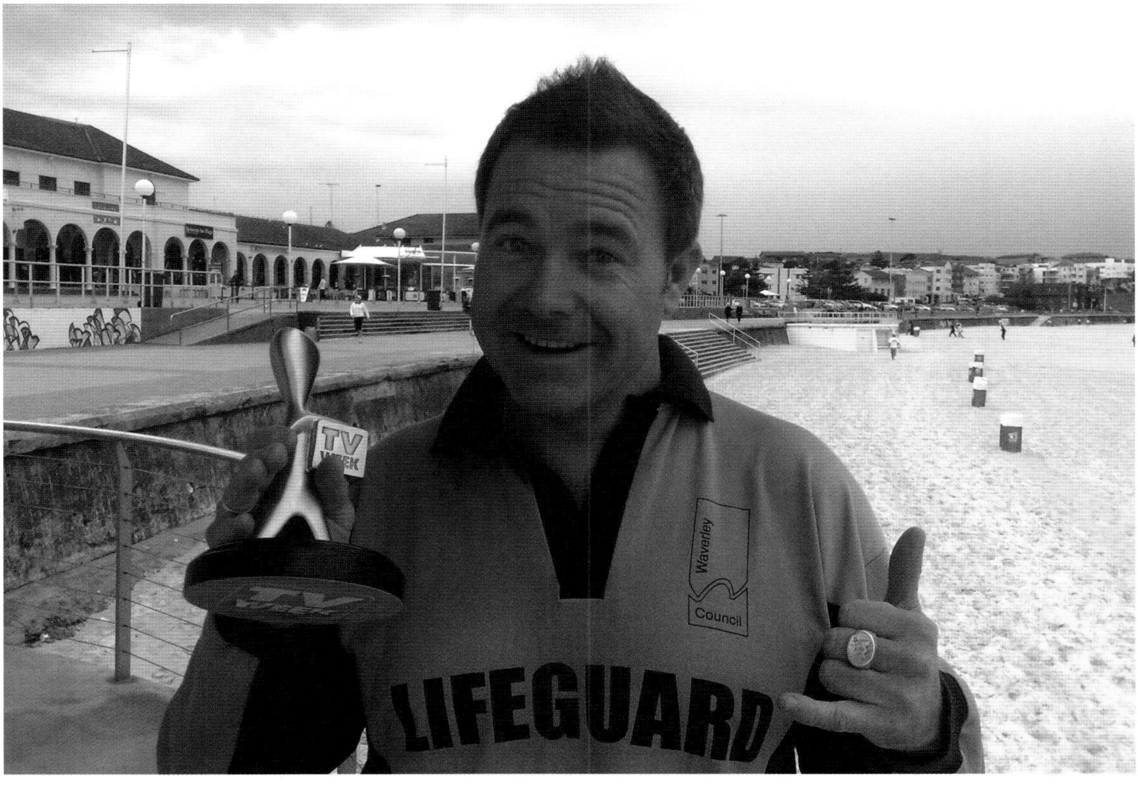

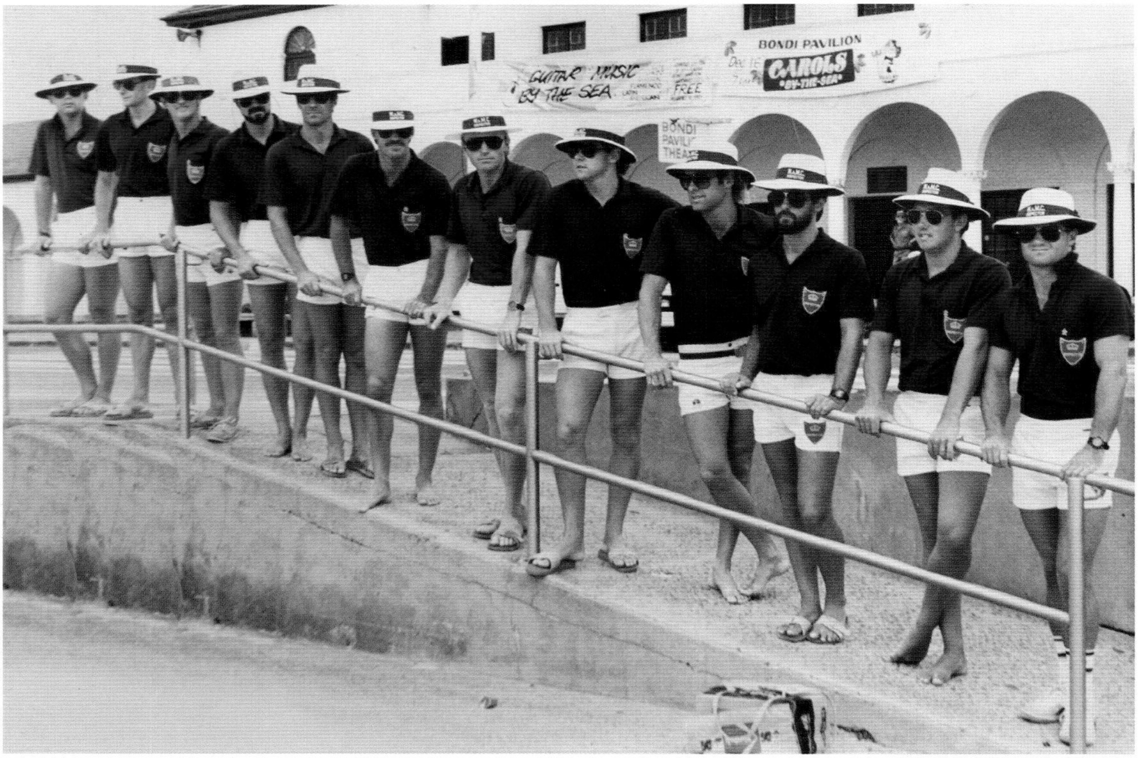

ABOVE Fashion has always been a watchword at Bondi. Beach Inspector lineup in the 1970s.

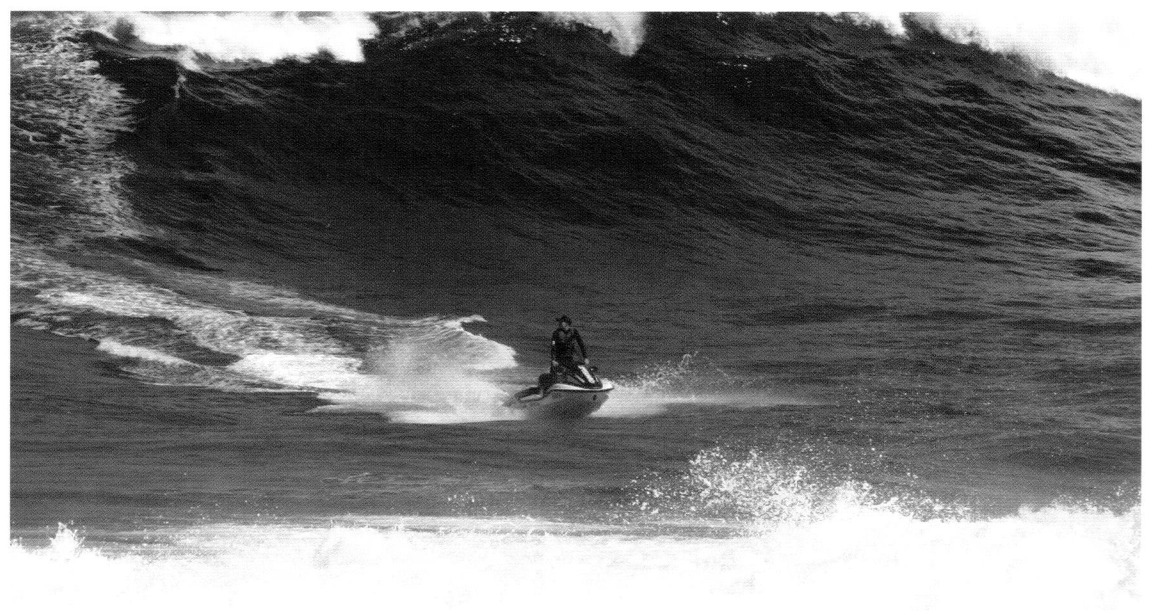

ABOVE In this kind of surf, the PWC's anything but a toy. Reidy running inside a major set of waves, centre Bondi.

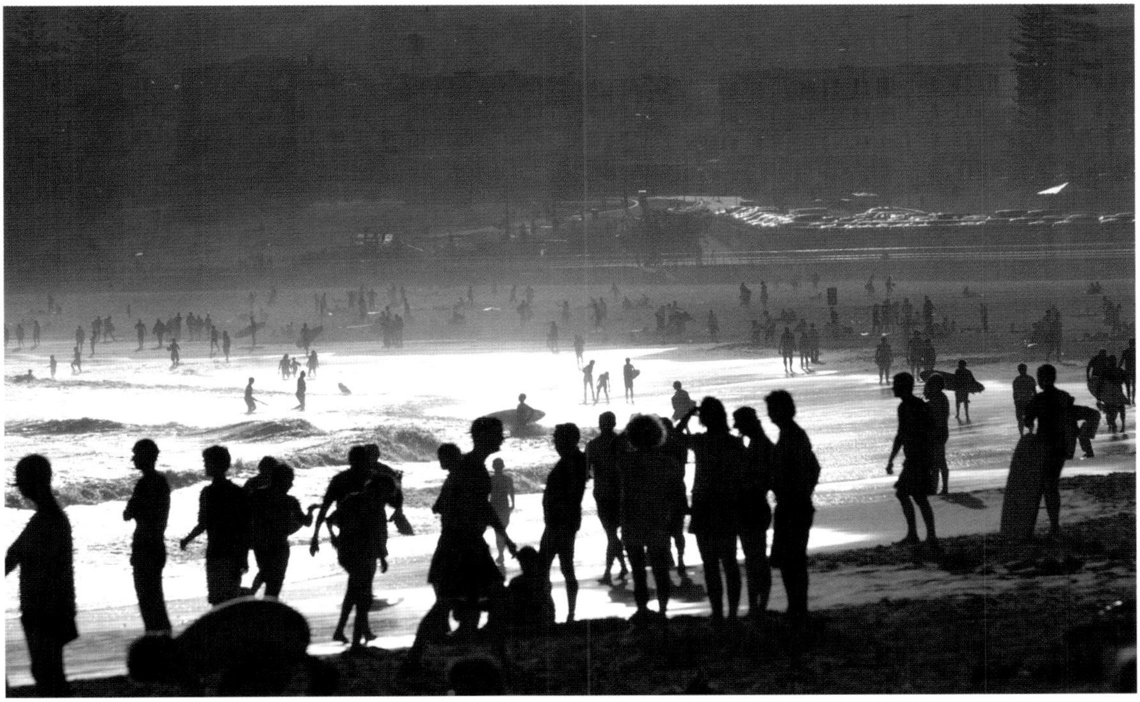

BILL MORRIS

ABOVE Those gorgeous after-work hours in midsummer—this is when all the big rescues seem to happen.

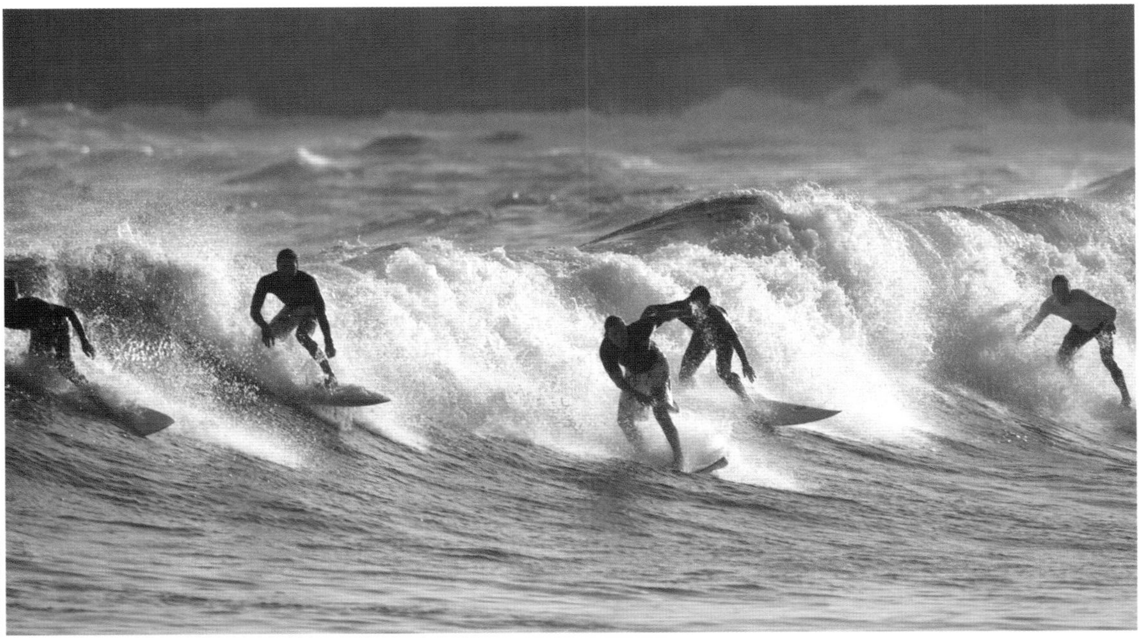

BILL MORRIS

ABOVE Normal surfing rules—give way to the one nearest the curl—don't always apply at super-crowded south end Bondi.

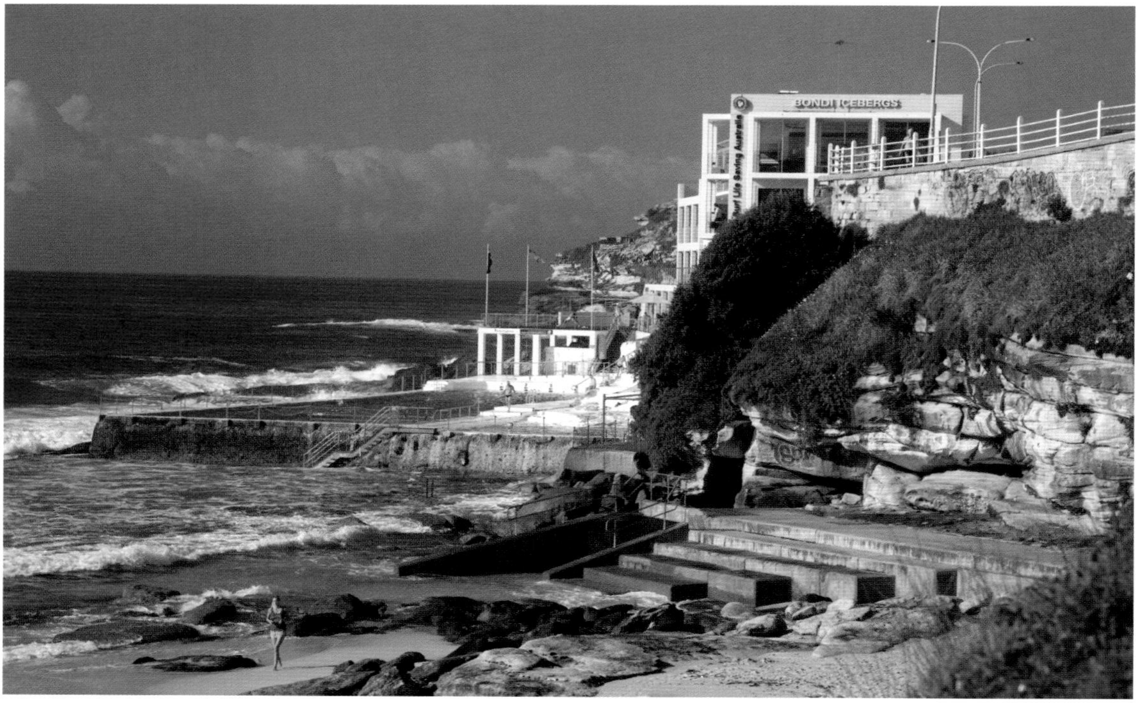

BILL MORRIS

ABOVE Bondi's got as many angles as it has people. From the southern walkway looking towards Icebergs ...

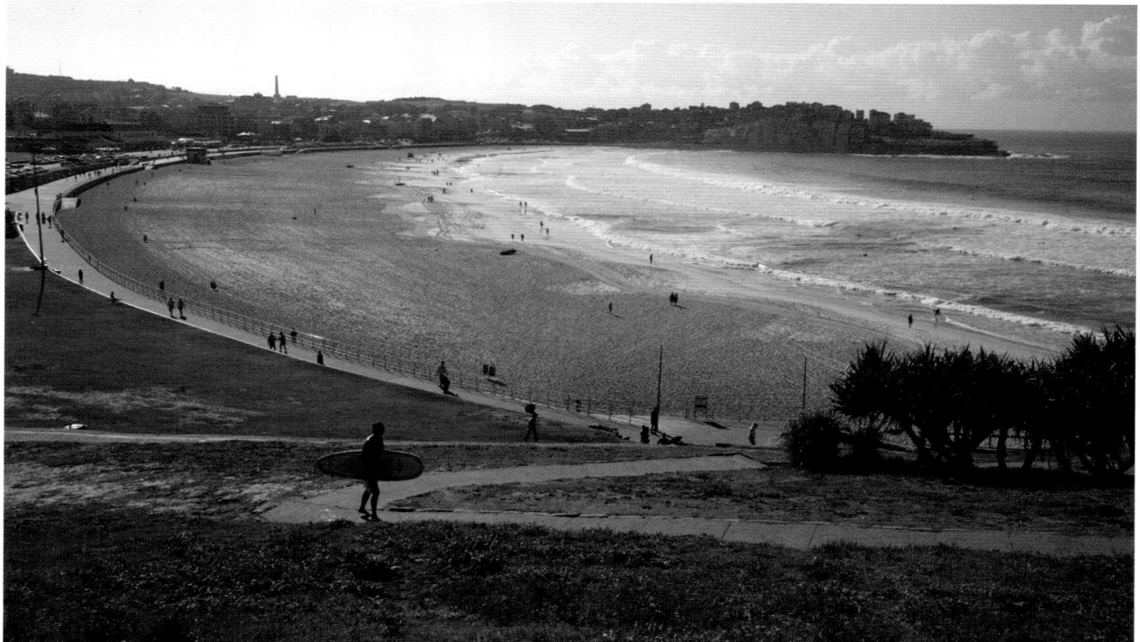

BILL MORRIS

ABOVE ... from high on the southern hill, that model's-smile arc of sand emerges ...

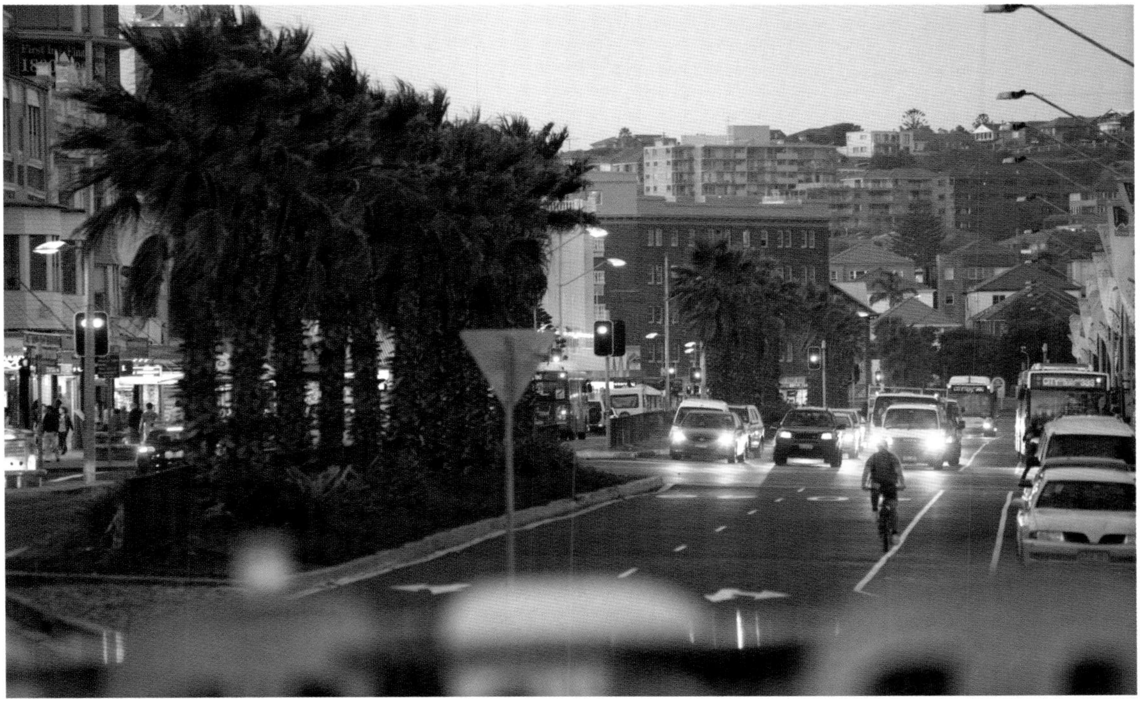

BILL MORRIS

ABOVE ... while behind the beachfront, Campbell Parade busies itself day and night.

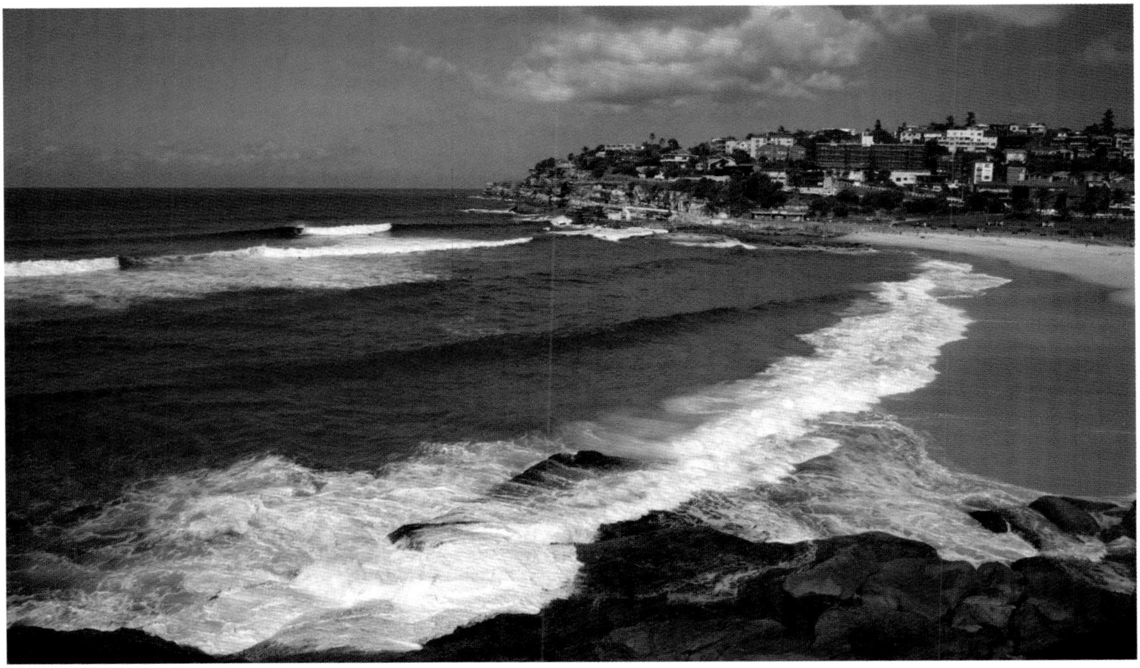

BILL MORRIS

ABOVE Bronte: a smaller, family-friendly beach, but still with its hidden dangers.

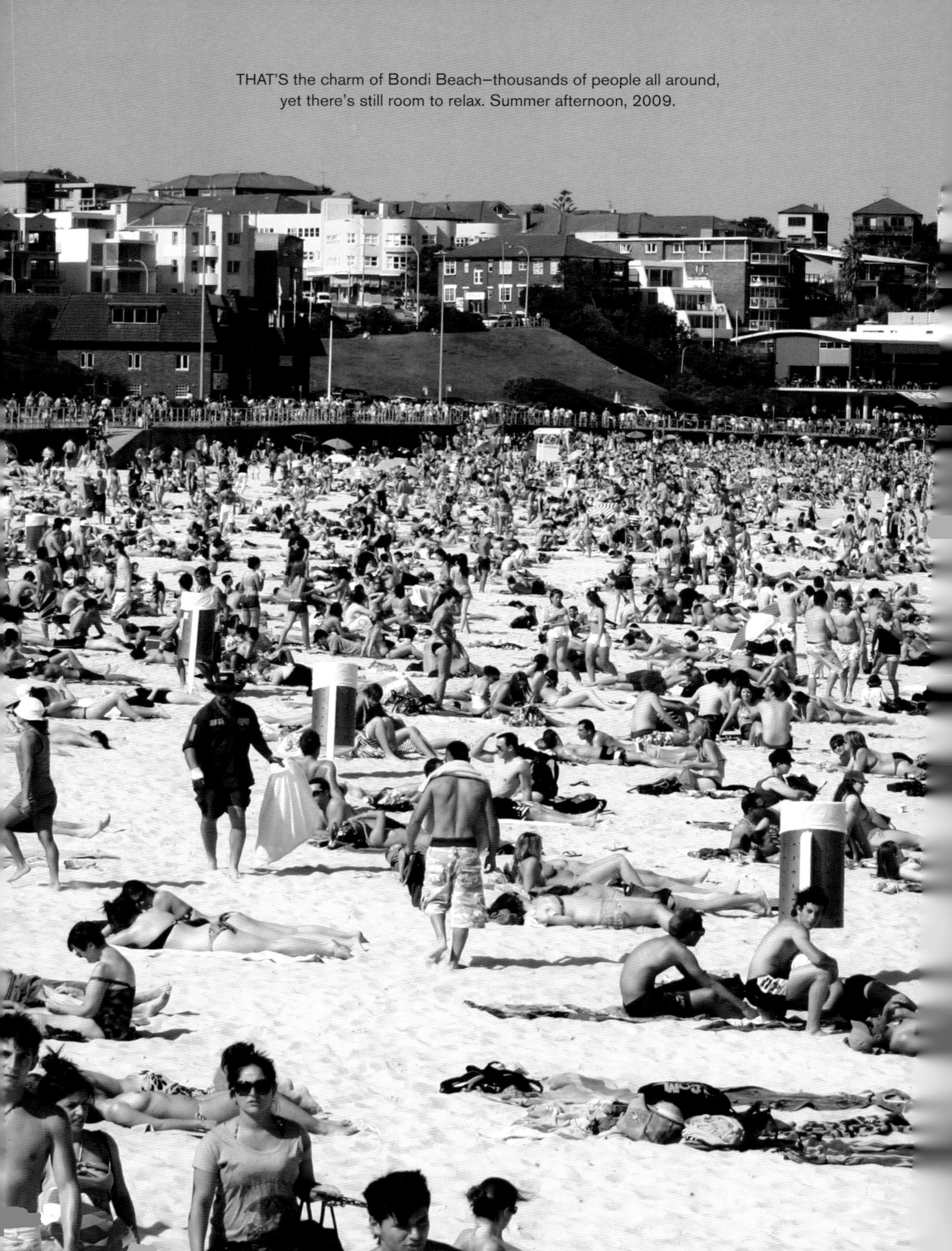

THAT'S the charm of Bondi Beach—thousands of people all around, yet there's still room to relax. Summer afternoon, 2009.

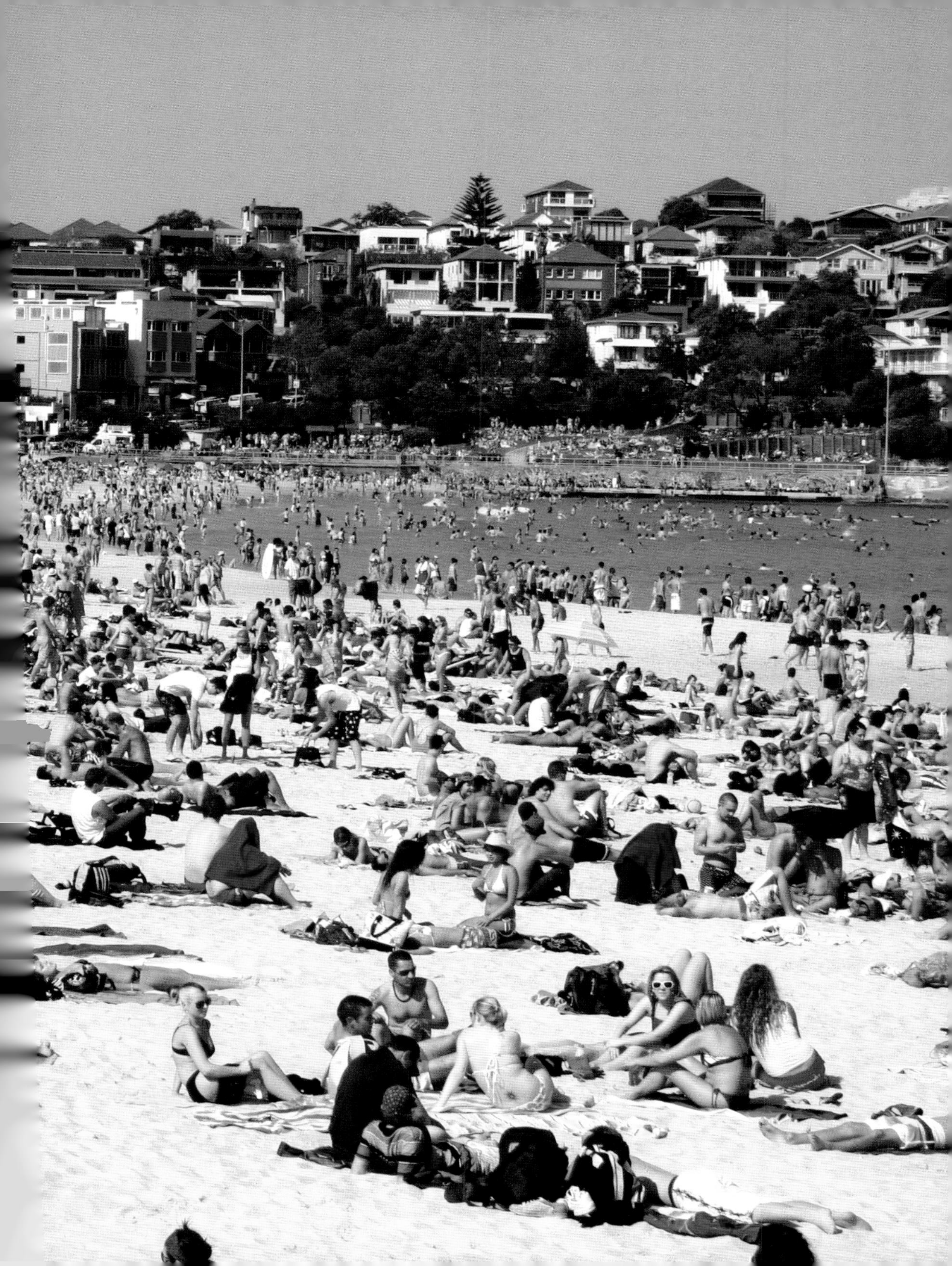

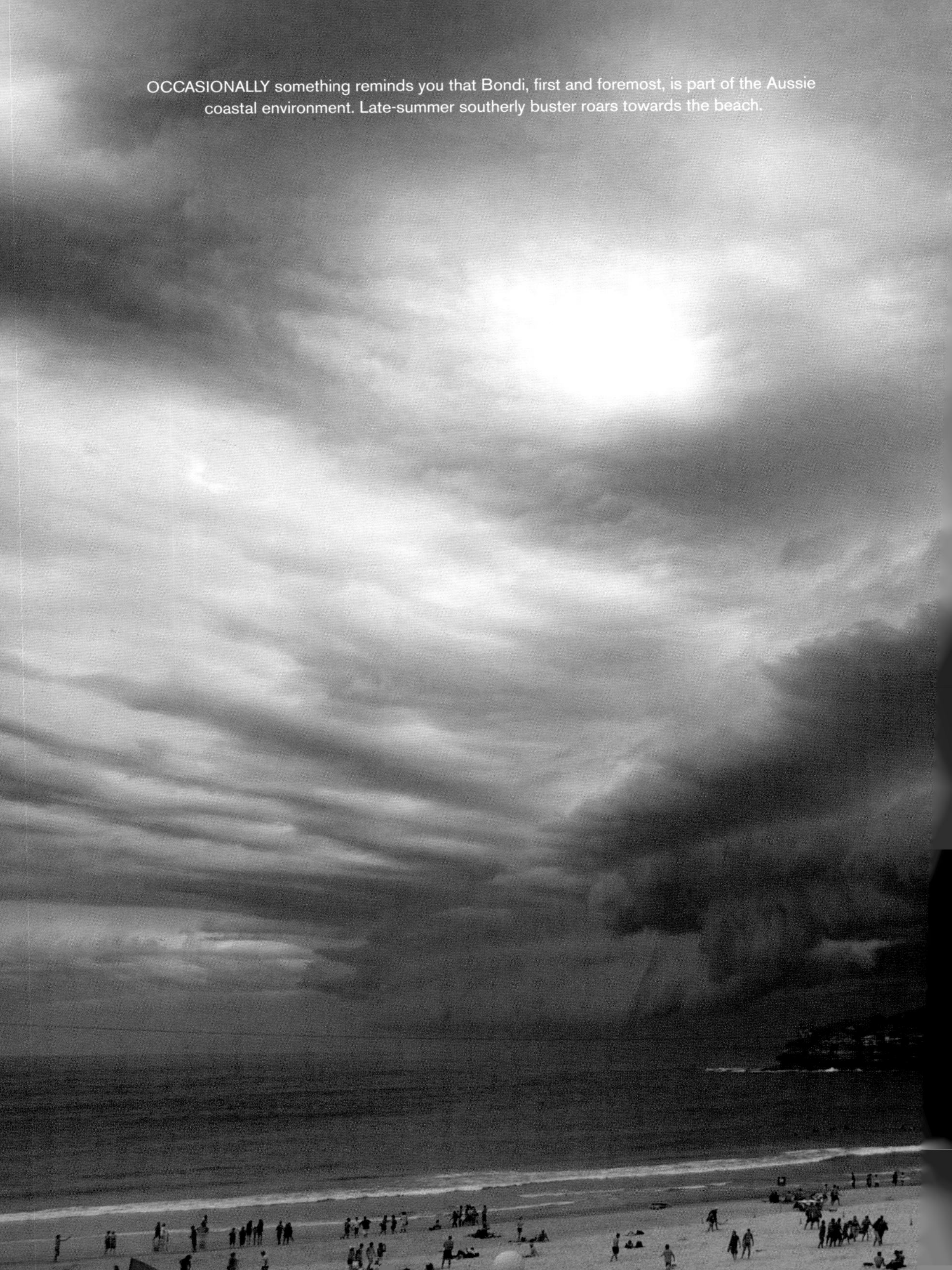

OCCASIONALLY something reminds you that Bondi, first and foremost, is part of the Aussie coastal environment. Late-summer southerly buster roars towards the beach.

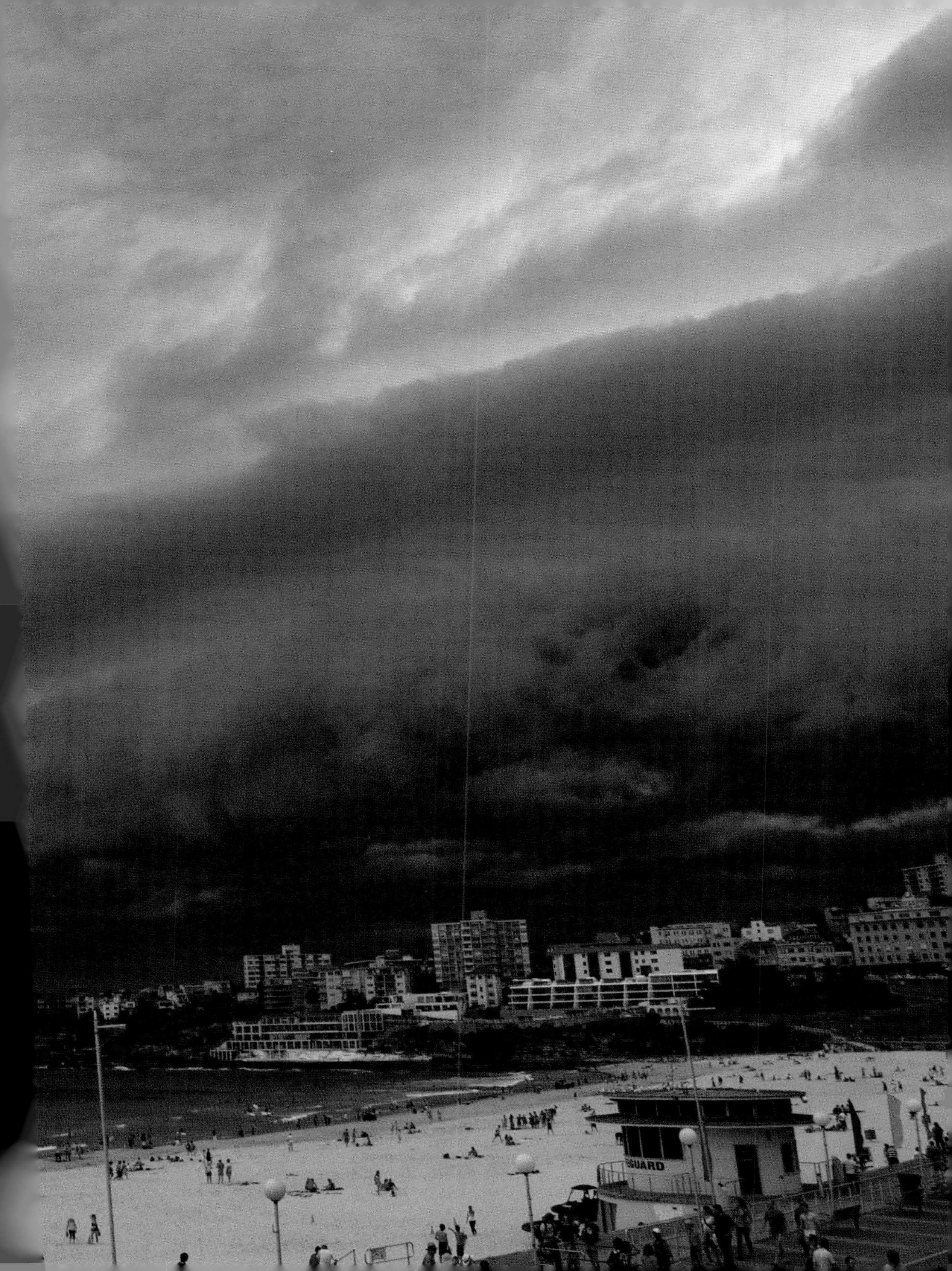
GUARD

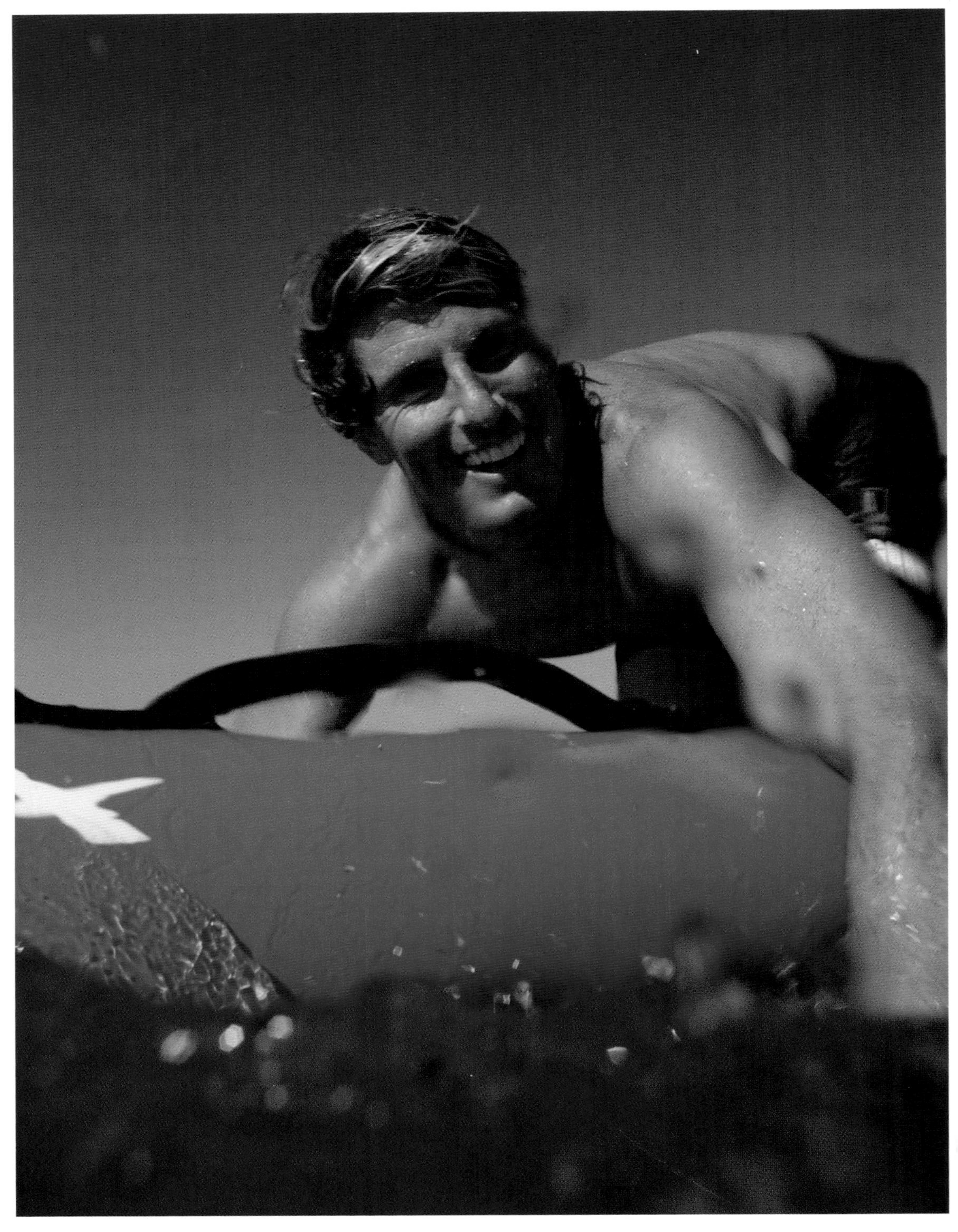

ABOVE So much of the job is about equipment. Harries gets a grip on the water and his board …

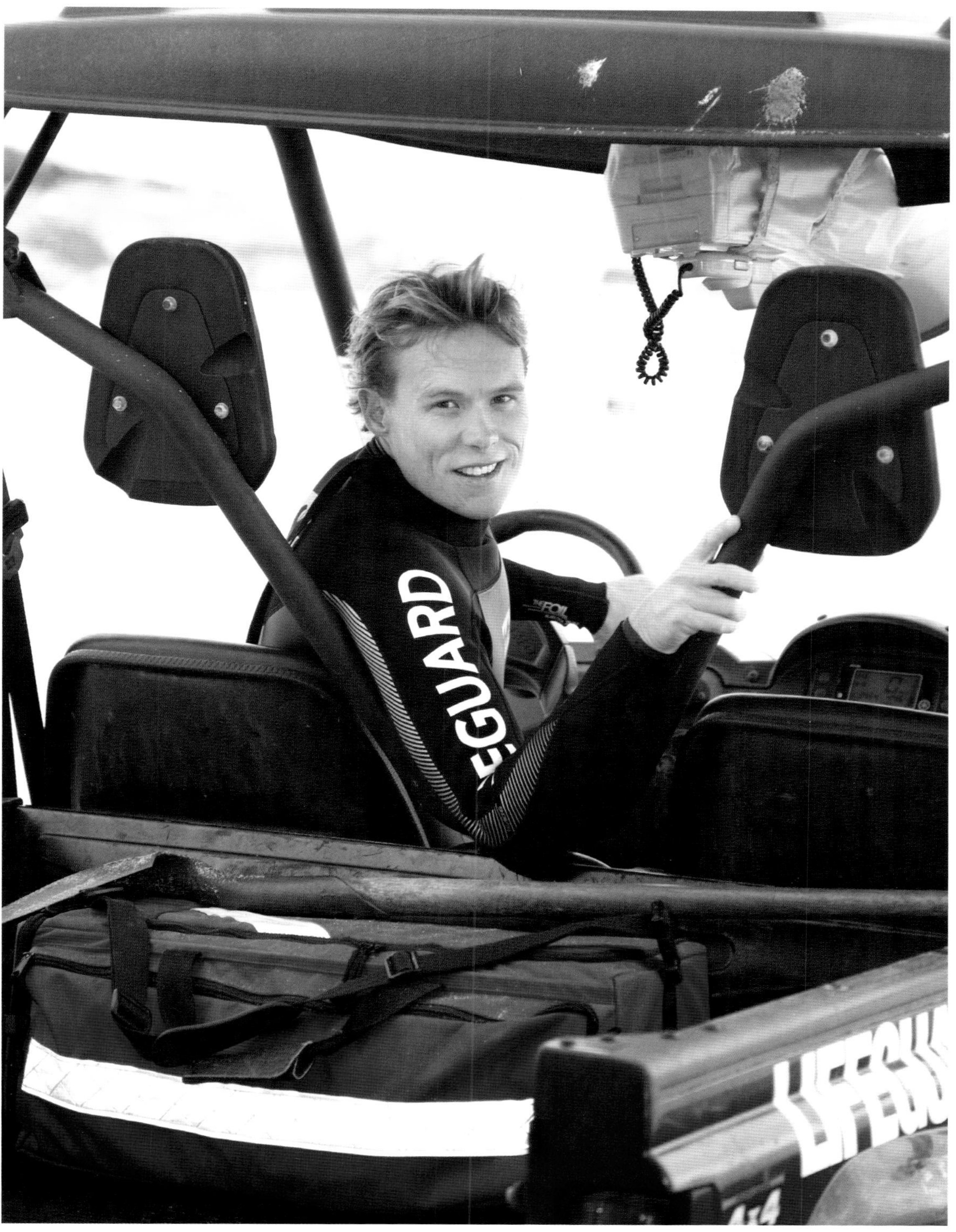

ABOVE … while Reidy, fastest rhino driver in the land, takes the wheel of his favoured machine.

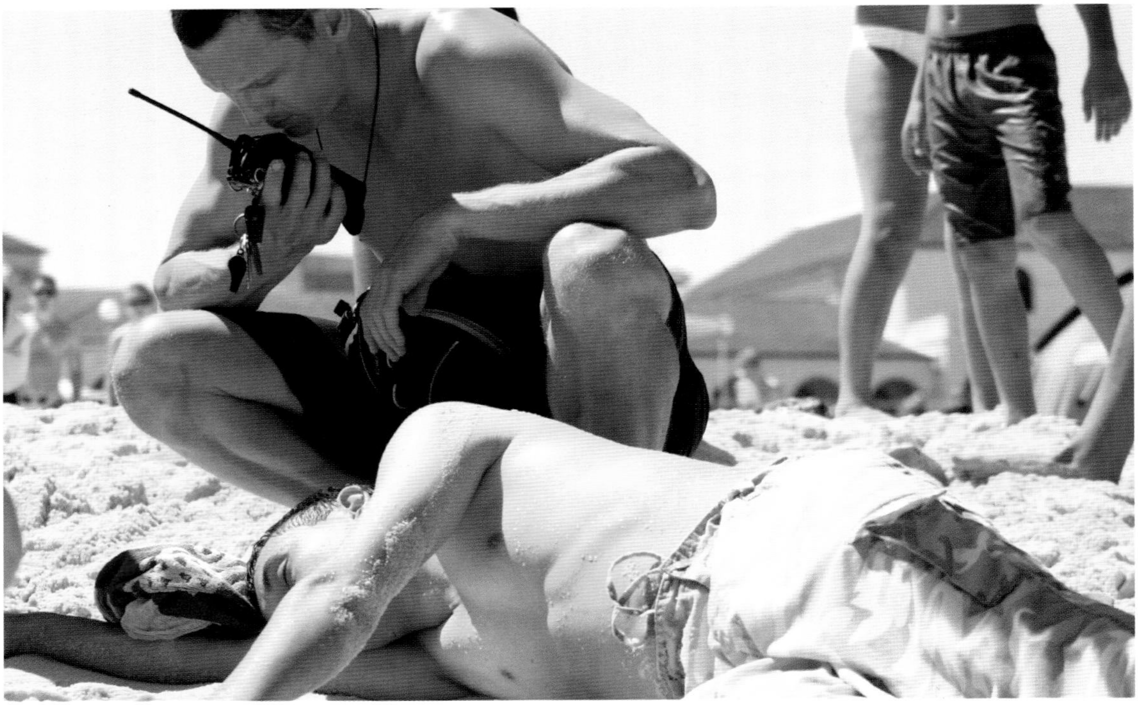

ABOVE Communication is of the essence. Calling in progress on a recovering patient.

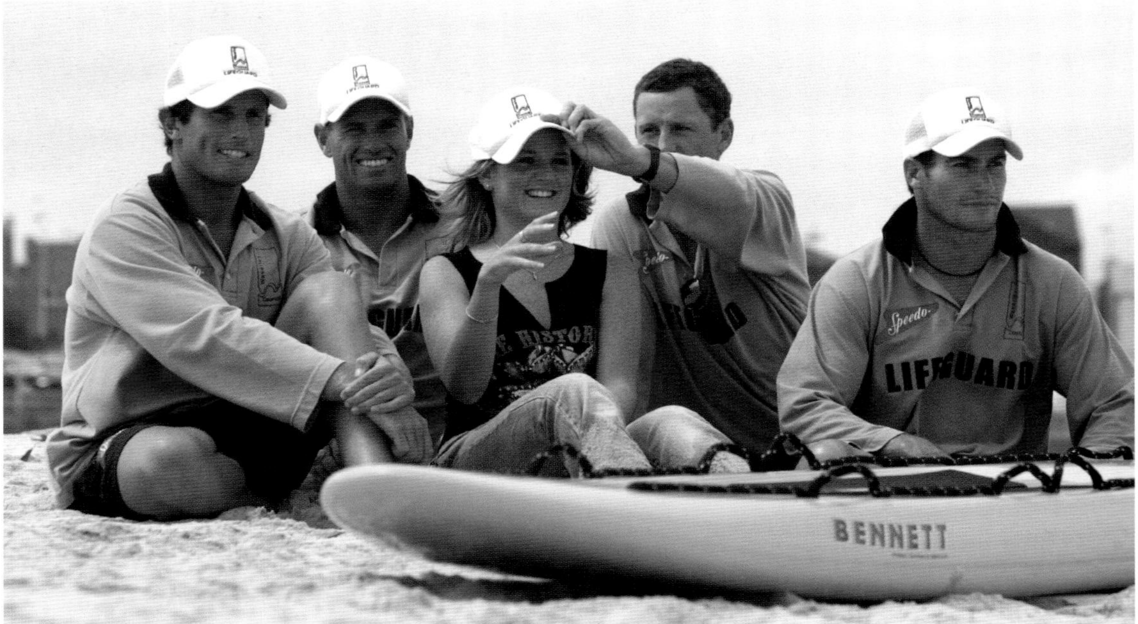

ABOVE She's still with us! Candice Tanne, drowned and resuscitated, post-recovery with a few of the team.

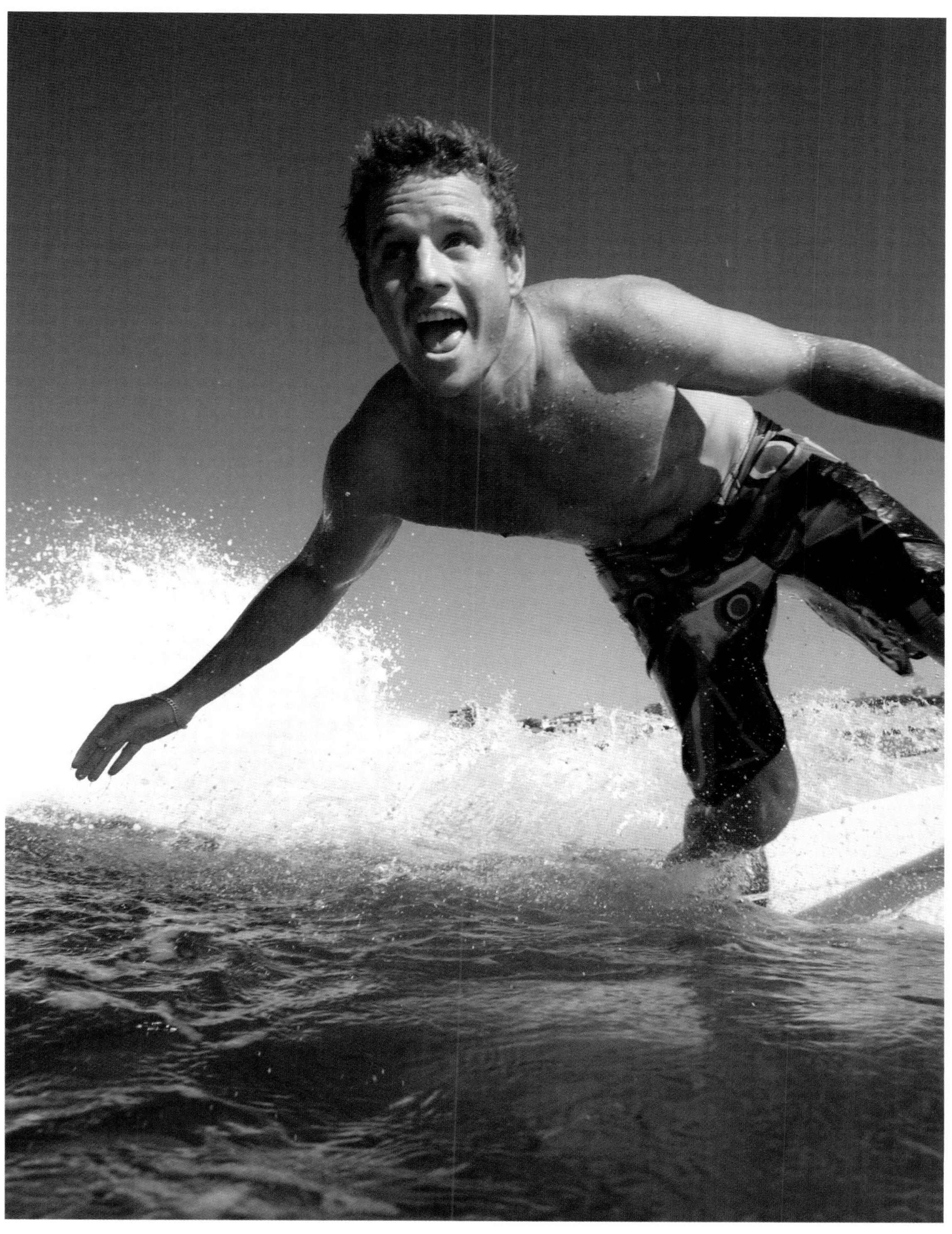

ABOVE In the face of this job, it's important to stay light of heart. Whippet playing in the south end shorebreak.

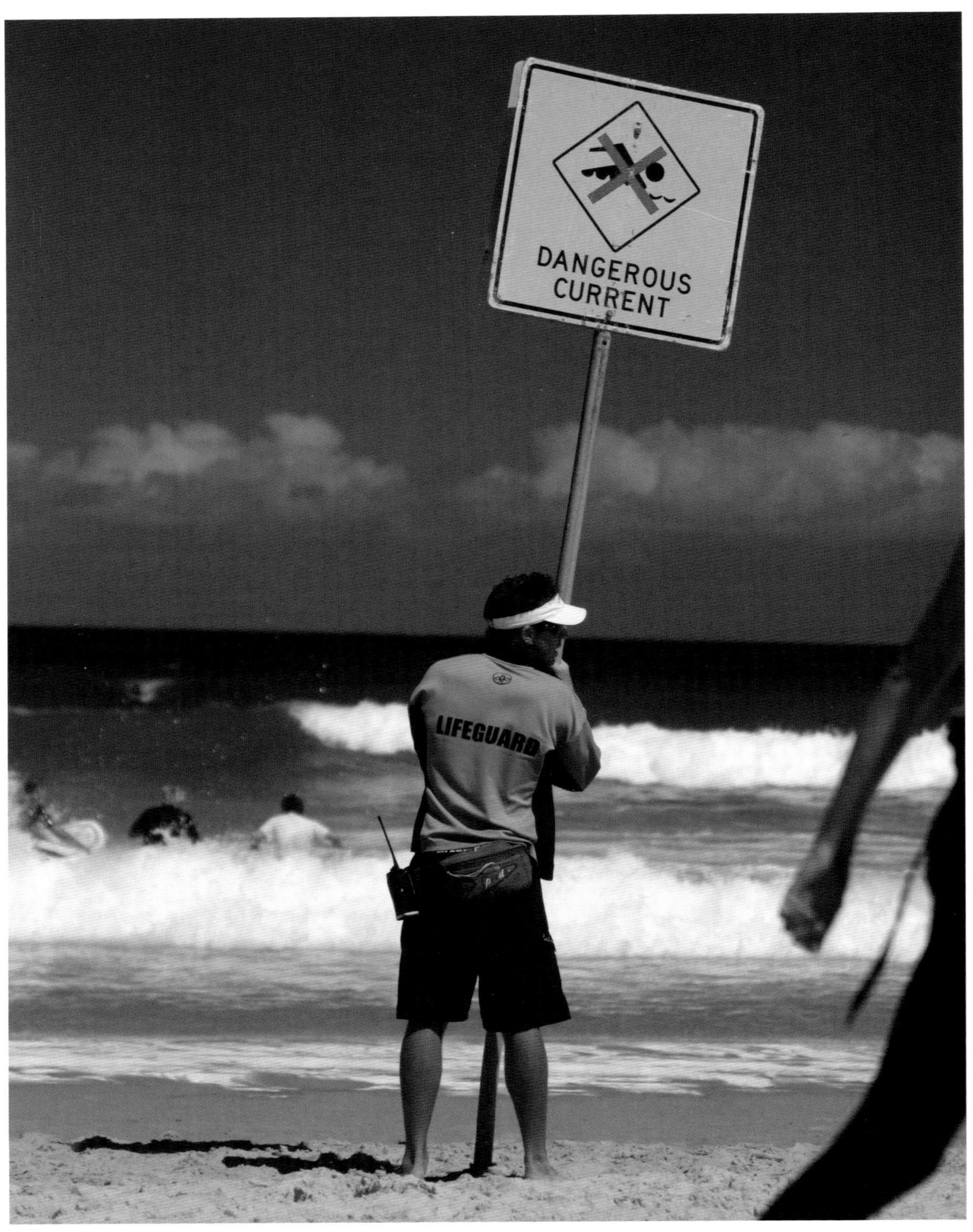

ABOVE The sign says it all. It's just a question of who's paying attention–and who isn't. Corey setting the ground rules at mid-Bondi.

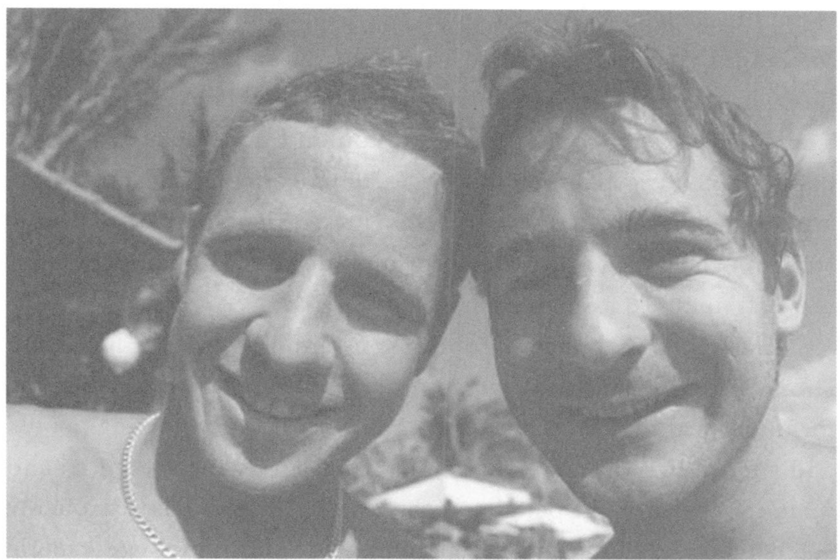

ABOVE Away from the pressure.
Bronte boys Whippet and Tom on duty break.

come, the swimmers on the fringe of the sandbanks would all be washed off into deep water. And then they were gone. As the tide began to drop, it just got crazier.

'We literally had bodies lying all over the beach,' Box recounts. 'Harries and me, he was looking at me swearing. Three or four of us were there all day just going, bang, bang, bang. We were trying to megaphone 'em out of the water, but there were 40,000 people on the beach and we just couldn't keep 'em out of this hole, it was impossible.'

The Black Sunday comparison kept coming up in Harries's mind as he sat in the tower, trying to direct the troops. He recalls: 'At that stage I'd done about 35 rescues on the board, and I was sitting watching 25 people drown at once. All Asians and Indians screaming for help. I've never roared so loud into the radio. The boys were doing everything they possibly could. They had ten on each board. The clubbies came to help and they couldn't understand what was happening. It was like watching an earthquake, a building crumbling around people. Amazingly we got 'em all in. Then there were people stuck on the beach and we had to provide resuscitation. The boys were all doing 35 rescues each.'

Harries took the jet ski out, just as another mass of humanity slipped off the sandbank and into the rip: 'Kerrbox was screaming for me. It was almost either us or them, cos if ten drowning people had got hold of ya ... so it was a fight for survival between us and them too. I had eight people on the jet ski, the ski was completely submerged and puttering back to shore, putt putt putt. I was a metre from the shore and I was yelling "Get off!!" The whole beach was watching. I knew I had to get 'em off so I could go and get the next group out of the rip. Some were getting on who were in trouble; some were half in trouble but half doing it for the thrill, they were hanging on cos they thought it was a joyride. I did a whip on the ski at probably 40 kilometres an hour, to try and shake 'em off.

'By 7.30 p.m. that day ... I don't drink much at all but at the end of the day I had a beer in my hand, reflecting on what we'd done.'

Reidy, in his first season on the job, was astounded: 'We were still doing preventative actions, stopping people from going out into rips, but ... It just felt like the tourist coaches were lining up in the car park and along the road, and the Japanese and Korean tourists were just lining up, walking off the coaches and straight into the rips, and we were bringing 'em back in and they'd walk straight back to the coaches. The jet ski did 70 rescues alone.'

'We were there for hours and hours,' says Kerrbox. 'It was the craziest day I've ever had—235 was a good number, but truly there were 250, probably more. I couldn't get out of bed the next day.'

It pointed out Bondi's biggest lifeguarding issue: pure crowd control. Kerrbox explains: 'The rip was close to the main set of flags so the majority of people were right there. You can't get 40,000 people into one set of flags, it's not going to happen. They're not going to walk down to the flags anyway; if you're down the south end and look out and it looks safe to you, you'll go out there.'

In the following week, with the beach set-up the way it was, Harries reckons they did another 1000 rescues. Yet somehow, no lives were lost, and he and the others remained on a high, even when not everybody they spoke to was willing to accept what'd occurred.

'I told one of the older lifeguards who'd been on for about 20 years what we'd done,' he says, 'and he didn't believe me. Which made me angry. Because those guys were all good lifeguards, but they did what they had to do to get by, whereas the guys now are exceptional surfers. They're taking off on 25-foot waves, or they're out there training every day. They've become the delta force of lifeguarding in Australia, if not worldwide. It didn't matter what a 20-year lifeguard had said to me. We knew what we had done and it was amazing.'

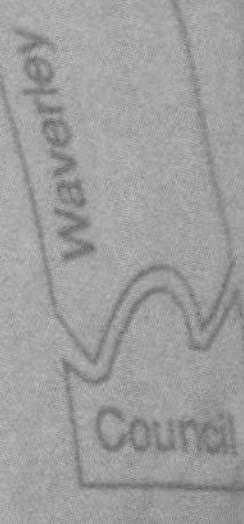

BILL MORRIS

Tom: The Student
(Tom Bunting)

'He used to be the quietest guy in the room,' growls Kerrbox. 'The whole first year he never said a word. Now he's the cheekiest bastard on the beach.' Tom Bunting laughs at this description. 'S'pose it's a case of growing into your own skin,' he says.

Each summer changes a lifeguard, and 2009's summer months seem to have caused Tom to relax. It's also provided him with a nickname—'Egg'. 'Must be comin' out of his shell,' Box chortles. Tommy looks as if he's about to say something he might regret.

Why would it come as a surprise that a lifeguard might be relaxed, or have a nickname? Perhaps because Tom Bunting is a step or two away from the classic Bondi lifeguard profile. Son of driven, professionally minded parents, he went to the exclusive, expensive Cranbrook School, holds a Bachelor of Science degree in biotechnology from the University of NSW, and is part-way through a masters' degree in chiropractic.

He doesn't need lifeguarding as a career; indeed sometimes he say he feels a bit guilty about the job, as if he's using it just to prop up his other life goals. But lifeguarding appears to fill another, more interesting place in Tom's head and heart—for him, it's a path to an old male virtue. 'I had worked in teams before but none had had the kind of camaraderie; the solidness between a group of guys like what we have now. We might joke about things, but when the time comes we all form a unit, and it's great to be part of that. You can't put a price on that. I think of some of my school friends who've already started out in their careers, they don't have that sort of bond with guys, it's priceless.'

Tom's a naturally quiet, controlled person whose face occasionally crinkles into a smile; when it does this, he looks like a different person. He's quietly spoken and highly articulate. There's a layer of something else, some intensity, beneath the dark eyes and quiet voice.

Perhaps that's not a surprise when you consider what his parents have done. In the late 1960s John Bunting, an Englishman in his early twenties, packed his bags and came to Australia ... by bus. John travelled all the way through Asia, down the barely formed hippie trail, though according to his son, he was never an actual hippie. Rather, he was that massively rarer creature of the time—a committed British surfer. 'He used to make his own wetsuits,' says Tom. 'He'd heard about Australia and about the surf here, and packed up his bags and did it. It contrasts a lot with what he is today. When he told me the story, I had a hard time believing it because he's very strict and regimented.' John got a job in a shoe factory in southern Sydney, but hardly stopped there. Today he is general manager of human resources at Mirvac Group, one of the country's largest property developers.

Meanwhile, Donna Parker, a Canadian girl, had finished university and spent two years living in Europe. In 1973 she read a *Time* magazine cover story about Australia being the Land of the Future, and flew here with the idea of staying two years. She and

John met in 1976, married a couple of years later, and Donna, who'd become a high school teacher, eventually pursued a law degree. She is now a principal investigator for the NSW Department of Education into sex crimes within the public education sphere.

Thomas John Parker Bunting was born on 22 September 1980, in Sydney, lived at first in Chippendale, then moved to Tamarama in 1982, after Donna had decided it was a great place to raise kids. His parents divorced when Tom was fourteen. He has a younger brother Alex, 24, and a half-sister, Isabella (his dad's child). Mum didn't remarry. Tom lives at his mum's house up the line of the Tamarama gully; aside from it being a nice place to live, it also saves him money. 'Dad lives at Mona Vale so I've spent a bit of time over there too,' Tom says.

> 'I had the best of both worlds. I could come down to the beach and level out, then go back to school and study hard.'

Tom's dad no longer surfs; instead he sails a boat he part-owns on Pittwater, the magical stretch of water not far from his Mona Vale home. His mum has never been super active around the beach, though she did always believe in the balance between beach and real life.

Tom and Alex didn't go down the Nippers road in the fashion of Hoppo and Box and the Carrolls. Nonetheless they spent all their days at the beach. The brothers are both extremely skilled bodyboard riders; Tom was a professional for a while, and still has endorsement deals. Most of the lifeguards are surfboard riders, which puts Tom right in the middle of one of the beach's great cultural clashes. Does he feel it? 'Of course. Every day. Not a day goes by when I don't get some sorta abuse for being a bodyboarder, to say nothing of "lidder" and things like that.' Tom is smiling, but not all that broadly. He says he doesn't hit back. 'Originally I was a surfer, I grew up around Bronte and there's a huge surfing culture here, I grew up surfing with Tom Whitaker and Kobi Graham. When I left Bronte Public and went to Cranbrook—and I dunno why—I started being more and more involved in bodyboarding, and it got very serious for me.

'But I don't retort back because I know they're just different forms of wave-riding. I ride a longboard and a shortboard … it's water off my back. They both have their strong points and I don't feel the need to defend against that every day. Sometimes I fire back if I think of something quick at the time. But I'm hopeless at arguing, I'm no good at writing off.' (Well, he is surrounded by masters of the art.)

Cranbrook, with its fees pitched at the scions of the squattocracy and their big-city big-money cousins, was a big investment by his parents: 'You sorta feel like you owe them a set of good results. But having said that, Cranbrook is a good school because of the calibre of students who attend … they were surrounded by a world I was very unfamiliar with in terms of wealth and possessions.

'But I had the best of both worlds. I could come down to the beach and become level-headed, then go back there and study hard. I don't think it was forced on me by my parents, it was a decision that I made. I could see the benefits of studying hard.' The bodyboarding contest circuit put pressure on his schooling, but in the end Tom managed a balance—he introduced bodyboarding to the school, where it's become part of the sporting program. Then came university. Not many lifeguards with tertiary educations, are there? 'No, there's not … which is another thing I get constantly bagged about, just adds to the list,' Tom laughs. 'They've got a lot of material to work with.' Nonetheless, he does get questions from the other lifeguards about various aspects of anatomy, and helps them where he can.

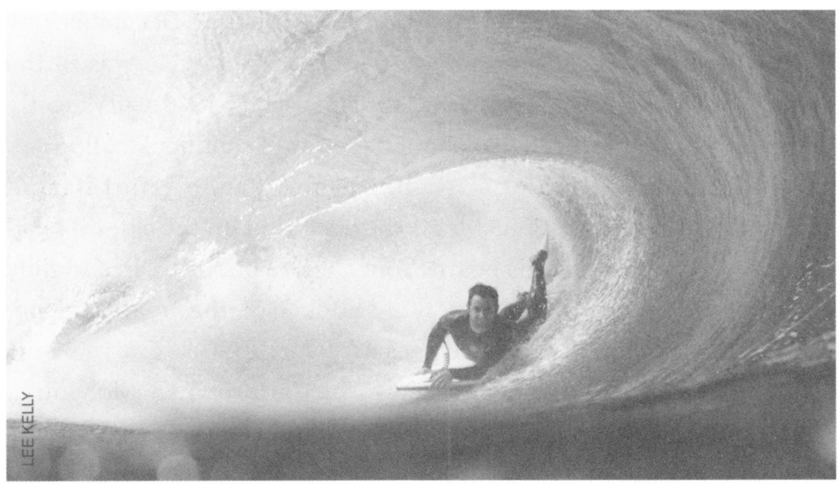

LEE KELLY

ABOVE Tom loves riding the tube. Down the south coast on a break.

Lifeguarding is something he'd always wanted to do, though it was a contrast with the futures being pictured by his Cranbrook friends. Tom worked as a lab technician for a while to help support his tertiary education, but found it boring, and remembered his interest in being a lifeguard. He put his head down and trained hard, spending months in the pool alone, unwilling to ask for help, and made it through the swim and M-course tests. He'd had several years of surf-tripping to Hawaii and Tahiti, which added to his skill level. He's seasonal, which gives him time for study, but works pretty much full-time through the critical summer months. 'It's not a chore any more. It's great. But it takes hard work. Going to Bondi is just another level. You're on your toes all the time. Everything I thought I knew about the beach, it was 5 per cent of what really goes on. Murphy's Law is the bottom line at Bondi, whatever can go wrong will go wrong, and everything else you could imagine after that.'

He first felt like one of the team on a dramatic December day during his first year, when there was a mass rescue. He was in the tower while Harries was out on the ski. The beach was already deadly thanks to the rip profile. Then about 5 metres of sandbank collapsed, and he could hear Harries screaming 'Third Ramp! Third Ramp!' Tom says 'I didn't think, I just ran.' Harries filled up the ski, Box had six or seven patients on his board, Tom got five on his own, and they got them all in. He ended up with Rookie of the Year, and got Lifeguard of the Year in his next season.

He was involved in the retrieval of the drowned Mongolian doctor in 2007, one of the team's hardest moments. Forty-eight hours later he was in the tower with Kerrbox, and saw three Korean girls being sucked out off the north end. Tom paddled out, pulled one girl up by her hair, and saw a blue face, a foaming mouth, no pulse. 'I don't even remember how I got her on the board. I think I basically picked her up and threw her on. Rod had started swimming, and he was screaming, "Get some breaths into her", so I did some EAR [expired-air resuscitation] on her. We got her back to shore, got the pads on her and got her back. She opened her eyes and coughed up a lot of water. Rod told me I'd screamed on the way in, "Please, not again! Not again!"' The girl walked out of hospital two days later.

Tom hopes to combine the chiropractic profession with lifeguarding, even if he is only part-time. He'd like to stay in touch with the camaraderie as long as he can.

'I hope I make Harry Nightingale age,' he says, on the beach one afternoon in mid-March. Tom's on between 3 and 7 p.m. today—the 'impact player' who can help relieve pressure on the crew, who've been there all day, when a Friday arvo crowd appears.

Tom drives one of the rhino buggies down near the centre flags, close to a rip that's just itching to pull an errant swimmer off his or her feet. Occasionally he presses the button on the megaphone: 'That bodyboarder just to the left … keep going across toward the sandbank … raise your arm if you feel you're in trouble.'

Then the *Bondi Rescue* fame-meter begins to tick. A bloke from Newcastle walks over with his newborn daughter—they're down visiting relatives for the weekend—and gets Tom to hold her while he takes a pic. Two girls from Queensland, who are fans of the show, want him to pose for photos. He engages them in conversation—'You watch every week? That's great! Good on ya'—smiles, shakes their hands. Quiet Tom is suddenly the PR whiz.

Unlike some of the boys, and despite being a contender for Bachelor of the Year, Tom has a long-term girlfriend, Claire Norman, who's a champion longboard rider. Claire's parents have a place up at Crescent Head and the pair go up there regularly on off weekends. It's a contrast with what most people assume about the Bondi crew's sex lives, given the clientele suntanning day after day at the beach. 'I'm not gonna lie to you, it's hard, it's in your face all the time and being a lifeguard I'm sure is an attractive thing for a lot of females,' he says. 'There's times when you could get away with murder. But it comes down to who you are as a person and what you believe in. I'm very happy in my situation … I just laugh at Harries, every now and then he utters these words of wisdom, ya know, "Tommy I really wanna be like you, settle down, go up the coast longboarding with my girl", and just an hour before he's been telling me about stuff he got up to on a surf trip that I didn't even know existed!'

This sounds a lot like a conscience at work—the same conscience that's got him through seven hours of study that morning, that keeps Tom wondering if he's almost too lucky to have both the beach and a brain. 'For me it's about a balance,' he says. 'Right now I feel content.

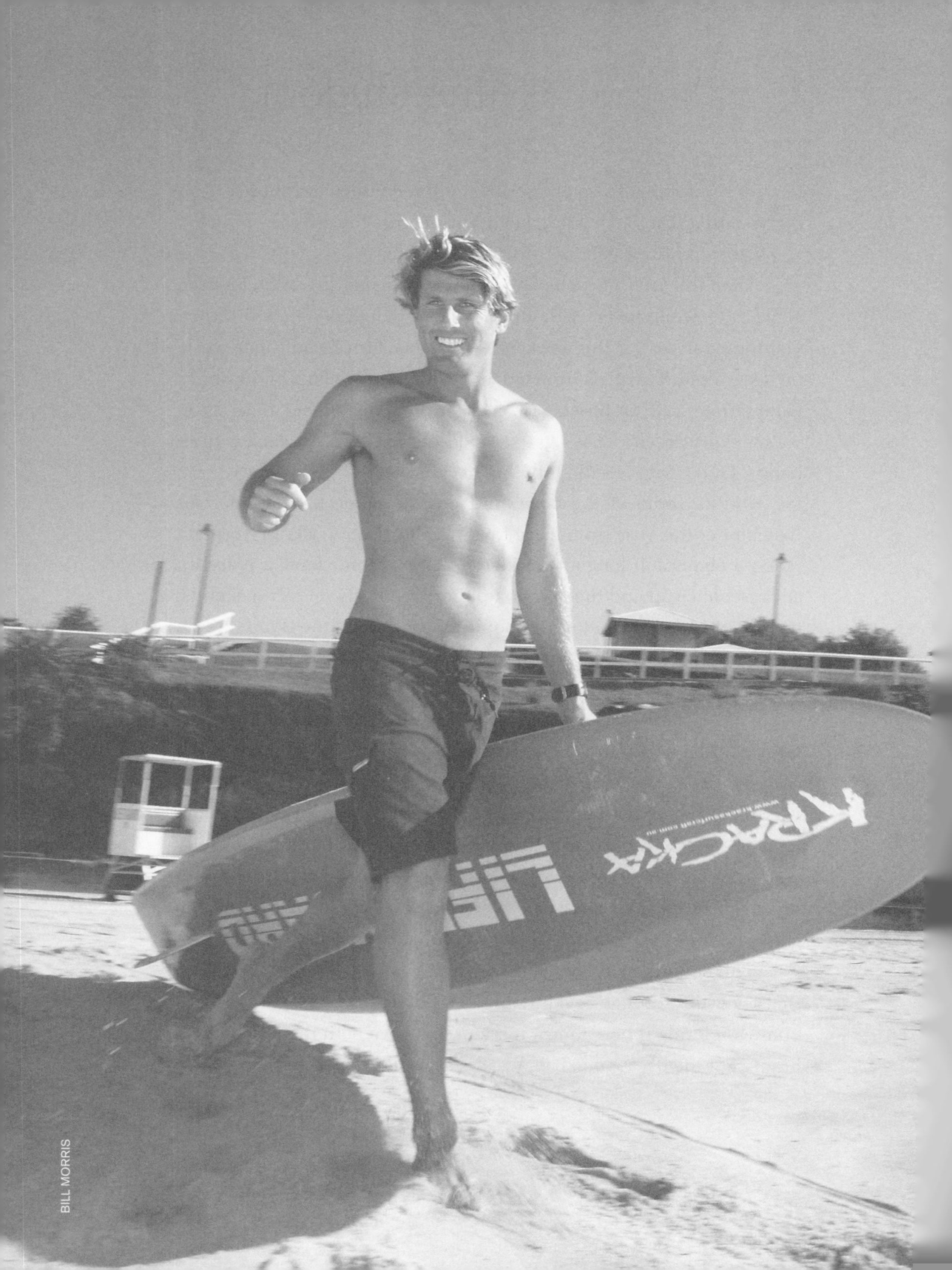

BILL MORRIS

Harries: The Extrovert
(Anthony Carroll)

'We've found what we are,' Harries says, an ever-present edge of amusement bubbling behind his voice. 'We're the product of our own environment. We were born down here and now we're doing what we'd probably do best.'

Anthony 'Harries' Carroll is lounging in a rickety wooden lifeguard platform wedged into the wet sand about 2 metres away from the Bronte low-tide line, watching his twin brother Sean surf the small waves off Bronte reef. Sean is a former lifeguard, a plumber by trade. 'He's quite bloody eccentric actually,' muses Harries. 'He can be down and out at times and he can be quite high. I tell him that he's good at surfing and at what he does.'

It's almost as if Harries is describing himself ... except even Harries might not be up to that task. To call him a larrikin or merely 'energetic', as many do, is to drastically undersell him; indeed, it's probably missing the point. He's possessed of an outsized life force which bursts forth in hilarious and unpredictable fashion. For instance, this is a man who's severely dyslexic, yet fascinated by the meaning of names. Including his own. 'Dad's right into his name history and I ask him what the Carroll motto is, and he says, "The Carroll motto is: We will bend, but we will not break." So funny!' The sonorous phrase cracks Harries up.

Later he tells his visitor, 'Bronte means "eye of the storm".' And while he's only half right on this score (in fact it's derived from Greek for 'the thunder-maker'), maybe that's where Harries and his fellow lifeguards are, in a way: right in the centre of their world, danger all around, but laughing all the same.

Anthony and Sean were born on 6 August 1976 in Paddington Women's Hospital to Mary and Ray Carroll, and were brought up in Clovelly, right on the water. The Harries nickname derives from a dribbly little Clovelly surf spot which the Bronte guys employed to make fun of the Cloey kids who came to visit: 'What's Harries like? Why aren't ya out there?' they'd tease.

'I think the women thought it was Dirty Harry,' says Anthony. 'It's stuck, I tell ya.'

The Carroll twins are tall, dark-haired, fit (Harries took out the 2009 Lifeguard Challenge by a sprint from Whippet) and very good-looking. As kids, says Harries, they were identical, though you can tell them apart a little more these days; indeed Harries does have slightly wilder eyes.

Their family background is a colourful one. Mary was a British subject of Egyptian, Greek and Italian descent, born in what was once Palestine, and had to flee the country after the creation of Israel following World War II. Australia was suggested, but to Mary's

RIGHT Harries is a natural board paddler; it won him the 2009 Lifeguard Challenge. Offshore at Bronte.

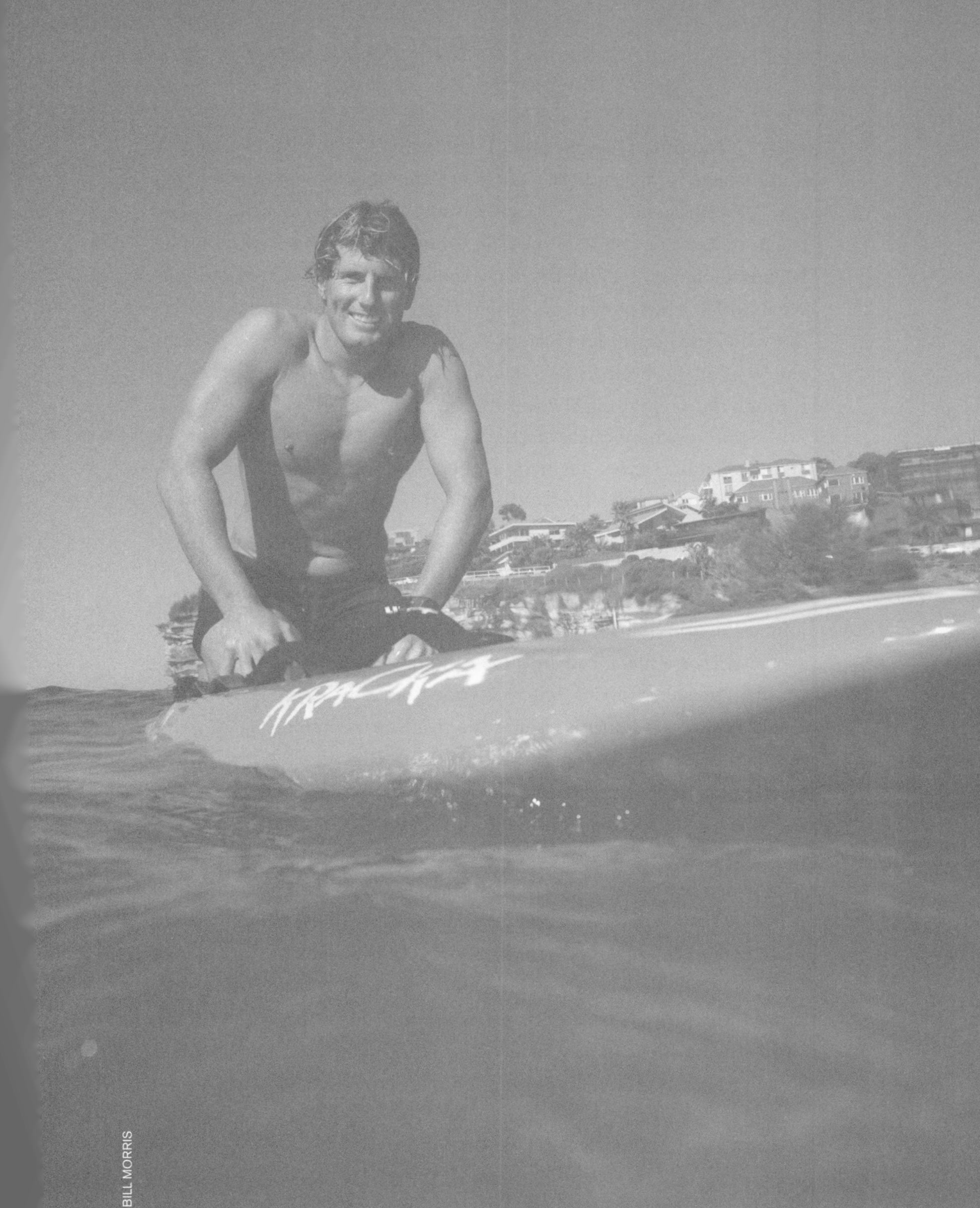

BILL MORRIS

parents it sounded like the end of the earth; they'd never even heard of the place. A year in post-war Greece convinced them otherwise.

Describing his mum, Harries says: 'She'd never been to the beach in her life, can't swim. First thing on arrival in Australia her friends took her to Clovelly. They took her into the water and she went under. Thus she never learned how to swim. But first thing she did when she had me and Sean was get the house at Clovelly, because she wanted us both to be champion swimmers, and to never go through the same thing she went through.'

Mum was previously married to a Greek dancer, and had kids at sixteen. Thus Harries has half-brothers Elias and Dimitri, and half-sister Eleni, whose son Brad is a lifeguard at Maroubra, five kilometres away. 'He's got exactly the same mentality as us,' he chortles. 'It's like we're three brothers.'

Ray Carroll was born in Paddington, grew up in Canterbury, joined the army and made sergeant before going to work for Qantas security. He's a black belt in three different martial arts forms and a jiu-jitsu master. Harries laughs every time he describes Ray. 'He walks under our house and hits his head on a wooden beam, tells me, "Mate I've been doing that for 40 years." How the hell does he do martial arts and still walk into this bit of wood every time?'

Dad also had a first marriage. His ex-wife Joan was wilder than Ray, according to Harries; he says, 'I just love her.' They had two kids who've led less fortunate lives than Harries and Sean. The twins feel sometimes like the lucky kids of the family—living on the coast, their parents knowing a bit more about how to make marriage work.

The Carrolls weren't well off, but where they lived has turned into Millionaires Row. Harries is very aware of this massive cultural shift—the sudden, almost shocking wealth, conferred by the near-accident of real estate, that has redefined Sydney's east. 'I was away on a trip with one of my mates and he owned a house on the corner above Bronte. And he said, "I dunno what to do, I've got this beautiful house but I can't park anywhere near it because there's so many people, I can't get all my kids down here, if someone offers me five million I'll take it." I thought, "Shit, five MILLION?" Two weeks later he says, "You won't believe what's happened, Lachlan Murdoch just knocked on the door and offered me seven million!" So he took that and went a bit inland and bought a house on a park about half the size of a football field for three million, and he's still got four in his back pocket! That's the changing trend.'

Harries and Sean grew up in their own little crew at Clovelly. It was a pretty much unsupervised existence, since their parents weren't really beach people; the older surfers, who often tend to form a sort of replacement family structure in beach society, ignored the grommets, so they did their own thing. The kids found their ways to neighbouring beaches like Bronte and Maroubra, and Harries has strong memories of Bronte's surfing elder 'Bluey' Graham and his sons Aaron and Kobi, who took him under their wings on surf trips up and down the NSW coast.

Both the Carroll kids had heavy dyslexia, could read a little bit but couldn't spell or write; they went to Marcellin College, where years before Rod Kerr had made himself a legend. 'School was interesting,' claims Harries, 'because we were so bad at it.' Despite this, they somehow passed the HSC.

At eighteen, Harries got a girlfriend, put on a bit of weight, and people started noticing. He thought to give himself a challenge to get back in shape. 'I thought: What are your strengths? Well, I'm good in the water. What are your weaknesses? Well, you're not fit, you might not handle an emergency too well, so throw yourself out there, get out of your comfort zone and challenge yourself.'

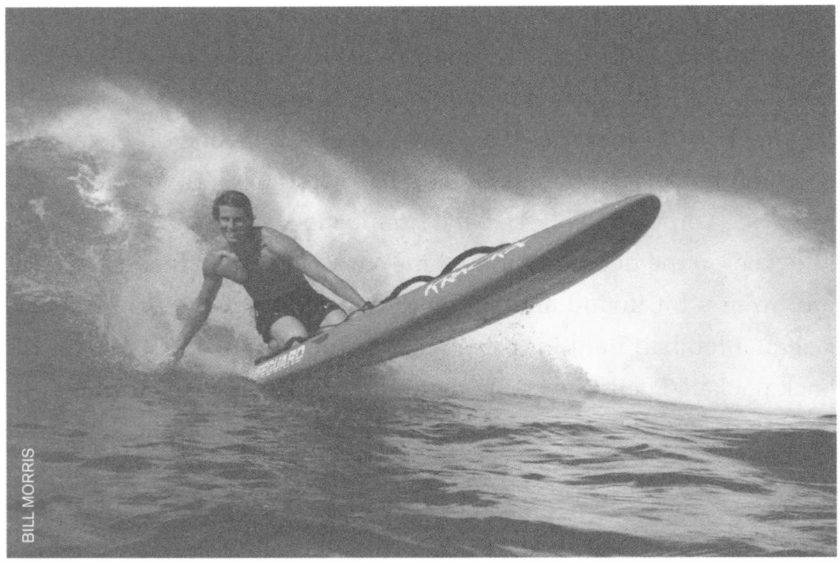

ABOVE Like all the crew, Harries loves a wave between rescues.

Encouraged by Kerrbox, he became a lifeguard in 1996. 'I was kind of one of the first young blokes. I used to really look up to George Quigley, blond, Greg Norman's double, the perfect bloke to look up to. You pick up things from older people and you definitely work out what's right and wrong but it takes time to sort it out in your own head.'

The dyslexia has left a legacy; it means that Harries is very visual, and has a very good memory. On his first day at work, he got down to the beach and headed out for a quick surf at the reef. There was a surfboat crew out; they caught a wave and as they hit the beach, they struck a member of another boat crew who hadn't seen them coming. The crew member was thrown from the boat; his ribs were crushed by the impact. 'Basically he landed in my lap. Back then the medical training was pretty minimal. I did remember one thing, if you reckon someone's been badly injured on one side, lie them on the other side so the blood doesn't flow into the lung. The bloke was fucked, the ambos got him and put him away. He couldn't do any functional movement of his arms for six months.

'Next day, it was flat. Sunny. A beautiful day, nothing happening. I took my shirt off and sat back in the sun and thought, "I'm in heaven!" Then I look out to sea and see this bloke on a board, way out to sea, waving his arms. I paddle out and it's a girl, an American girl. I'll never forget it, she had mental problems and she was trying to commit suicide. She's saying, "I'm trying to kill myself but I just can't do it! I'm trying! But I used to be in the American swim team and I can't seem to manage it." There is a local mental ward at Bronte just up the road and she's done a runner and tried to neck herself. So I get her on the board and start paddling in and she falls asleep! I've got no idea what's going on. She's asleep on the front of my board and there's the doctor from the place up the road waiting for me on the beach.

'From that day on, for some reason, all the lifeguards say I generate every nut. They say a nut knows a nut and I draw the nuts to me. They see my eyes and they're drawn. I always say, "Hello fellas, how are ya?"'

Watching him at work is intriguing. One day at Bondi, while he and Kerrbox are on duty, a swarm of bluebottles cascades through the mid-afternoon crowd. Bluebottle days are the worst, most irritating days in a lifeguard's working week. There's almost nothing you can do about them, in fact, and without a full-beach PA system to warn all the swimmers at once, they can only watch the queue of stingees grow longer.

'Everyone has their time in the sun, and as long as you help others and give back a bit, you've done well.'

Box sits and tries to stay out of the action, while Harries fields the requests. 'Santa's Little Helper's here for you!' he tells two attractive girls; they grin up at him like they've heard a few lifeguard lines before. 'For God's sake!' he tells one group of Korean tourists, 'the whole family's up here!'

He really enjoys the communication. 'Coming out of having dyslexia, this is where I've been able to come more into myself,' he explains.

As it is, dramatic situations follow him everywhere. He tells a story of his flight to Bali in 2008: 'This bloke walks up the aisle past us and he smashes into the side of the chair and falls over, eyes rolling back in his head. I strongly thought he was dead. Just jumped up straight-away.' The guy was heavily dehydrated and Harries got him on electrolytes and let the attendants take over. Then went and kept drinking. 'The captain sent down a bunch of Krispy Kreme donuts and four vodka lime and sodas ... I was just like, this is gonna be the best holiday of our lives.'

Harries worked for a while as a Qantas flight attendant, which gave the incident extra heft. 'I was dealing with flight attendants who'd been there for a month, I hadn't flown in cabin crew for six months but I remembered where all the equipment was. I get really stoked with shit like that!'

He means, he likes being effective and competent. You wonder if, like a lot of kids with learning difficulties, Harries might've felt pretty incompetent at times at school, and makes up for it in the world he's made for himself in lifeguarding.

In Bali, he ended up teaching Kris Yates, a former Australian board paddling champion, how to surf. Yatesy was asking, 'What do I do if it tubes?' Then he'd paddle out and start asking Harries, 'What are those things releasing in me, making me feel good?' 'Endorphins!' Harries told him. Later Yatesy said, 'I've got that bubbly feeling again!'

'If there is a God,' Harries says, 'he's given me the opportunity to help people.'

Harries reckons he's set himself the ultimate goal: He wants to be a lifeguard to the age of 63. If he gets that far, he'll have lapped Aub Laidlaw. 'I reckon if I last till 63 I'll have done exceptionally well. I'll be the longest standing lifeguard and I wanna give all those life experiences back to the other lifeguards. Everyone has their time in the sun, and as long as you help others and give back a bit, you've done well.'

wild stories FROM THE SERVICE

The guy with the suit

ON THE BEACH at Kuta, during the 2008 Bali Rescue sessions, the crew notices a man in a full business suit, complete with umbrella, as if he's on a London street. This is an unusual sight, so they keep watching; fortunately they do, because the man calmly walks down the sand and directly out to sea towards Java. He keeps going until it's clear he's intent on drowning. The crew leap in and chase him down, hauling the man in the suit back to dry sand, where he evinces no real explanation for his actions—just heads off to go about his business. The lifeguards still have no idea what he was really doing, or what subsequently happened to the man in the suit ... but at least he didn't die on their watch.

The other guy with the suit

DOGS AREN'T PERMITTED on Bondi Beach, and while it's not a mega-priority for lifeguards, they'll do their best to help out their council-ranger colleagues, which is why Kerrbox and Harries set off down the beach one morning in a rhino when they spot a man walking his hound near the water's edge. As they get closer, they see the man is perfectly attired in a well-cut suit, right down to the three-button jacket and shiny shoes. Of course, they assume, this is a gentleman; perhaps he just doesn't know about the regulations regarding dogs. They pull up next to the besuited one, and Box politely explains the situation. The man looks them both up and down and replies without preamble, 'Get fucked!' Harries recalls, 'We pretty much fell off the bike laughing.'

The Mongolian doctor

MID-AFTERNOON ON AN intermittently cloudy day in January 2007. Tom, still fairly new to the job, spots what he thinks is the top of a head, in the rip at the south end. Reidy thinks he saw something as well and goes out on a board to look around. Tom calls for help, and by the time he refocuses the binoculars, the object has vanished.

It's all so indefinable. Surfers who've been in the area, within just a few metres, say they've seen nothing. Doubt circles the search that then commences; it's a crowded summer afternoon at Bondi, yet the lifeguards neglect everything else and search for the mirage for 45 minutes—a long time when there's 30,000 people on the beach. They find nothing. Then, just as the day is coming to an end, a kid comes up and tells them, 'Dad is missing.' Reidy and Tom immediately know what it means.

After another, shorter search, they find the body and bring it in. The victim turns out to be a doctor from Mongolia, a recent immigrant who's been in Australia less than a week. 'It was terrible,' Tom recalls. 'Mum and kids were on the beach right there. We can't pronounce him dead, so we put the pads on and commenced CPR, even though we knew he was dead. Kids were screaming, the mum crying, all were praying. There was a big crowd. Luckily the police were there and helped keep 'em back.'

Tom still speaks of this day as a mystery that might be able to be justified, but never solved. How a person will be there, then slip, then gone. How many times has it happened in the past? How many times will it happen again? He tries not to think of the what-ifs.

The great white

LATE ONE ARVO in December 2005, a hundred people are standing on the cliff above Mackenzie's Point at Tamarama, and according to Harries, they're 'screaming like monkeys'. The reason? A 4-metre-plus great white shark is cruising casually down the point. Its fin is sticking out of the water like a piece of furniture. The shark, first spotted at south Bondi, sends the cliff-watchers into a panic on behalf of a range of water-users—a spearfisherman, surf-ski paddle trainers and swimmers—who can't see it and for the most part have no idea what's happening. Harries takes a jet ski out to chase away the shark, and is blown away by the encounter. 'I wasn't scared, I was just in awe,' he tells a journalist at the time. 'We're in its backyard, you kind of respect it ... This thing was the king of the ocean.' The shark is gone by the following day, as far as any lifeguard can ascertain. It's a reminder of how little anybody knows about this coastline and its inhabitants.

The Tamarama hero

SEAN CARROLL HAS quit the lifeguard service now, but over the years, he and big brother Harries have done some big rescues together; at least one of those has an odd postscript.

'We had an American bloke, he was at Tamarama off the rocks and he was yelling "Help, help", but not really loud,' says Harries. 'It was one and a half metres of surf, not really big; he was big though, probably 100 kilos. It took us ten minutes to get him out of there, then Whippet and [fellow guard] Sam Marshall came out from Bronte, and we finally got him round to the beach. Near the end, one of the young clubbie blokes came out to give us a hand. We thought nothing of it.

'Then Whippet and I and a couple of other blokes went to an Aussie surf club championships. We're sitting round having a burger, and they're giving out an award for Australian Lifesaver of the Year, the most dangerous rescue in the most critical situation, and they've called out the young clubbie bloke who assisted us.

'He assisted us for about 3 metres. So it kinda ... It's kinda sad. I know the bloke really well, and I said, "Mate, you must be embarrassed." But at the end of the day if you look each other in the eye as lifeguards and say "How much fun did we have doing that?", it counts for a lot more than an A4 sheet of paper saying you're a SLSA hero. It means a lot more to us just to say to each other, "Good work".'

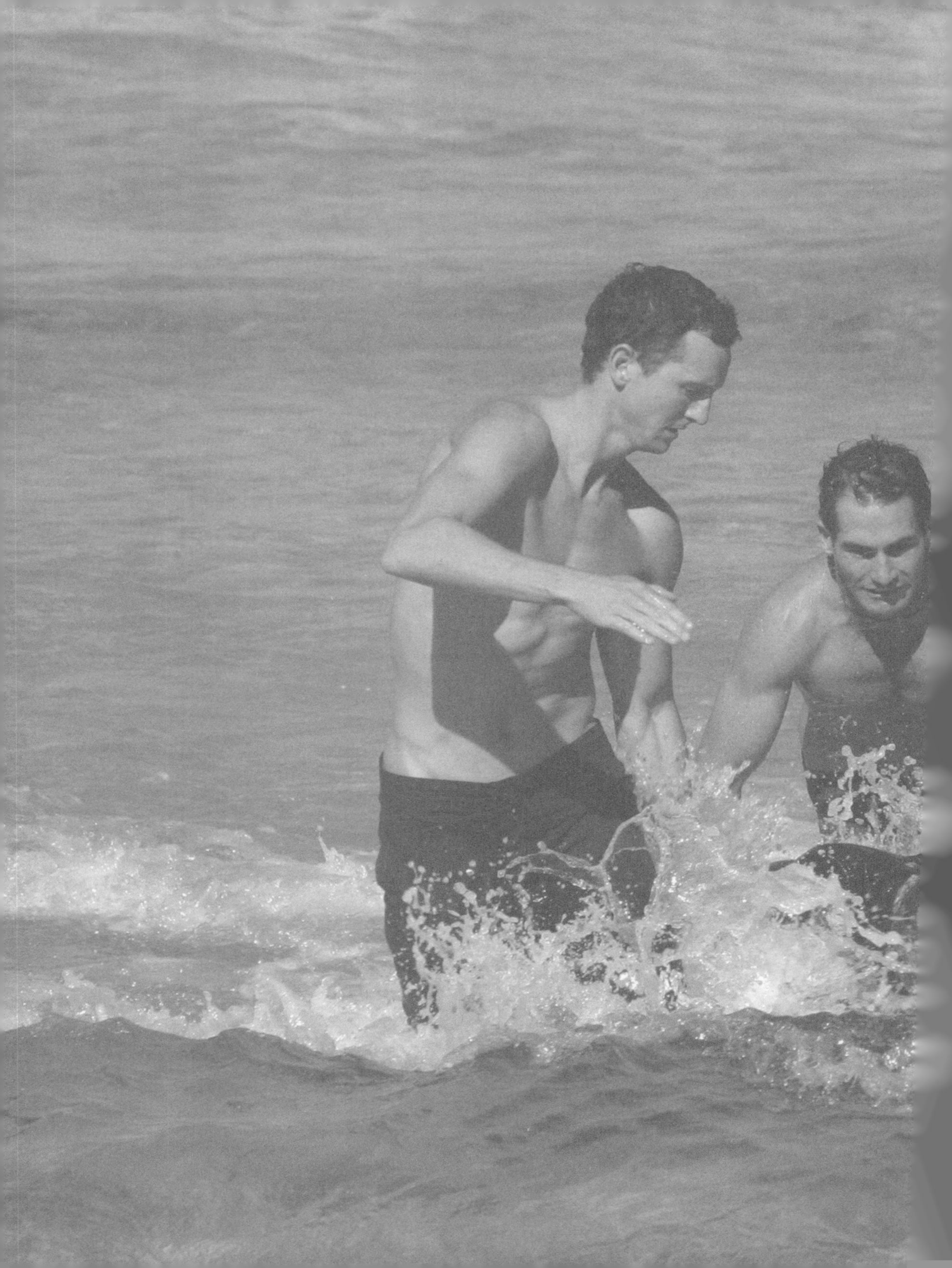

6
THE RESCUED

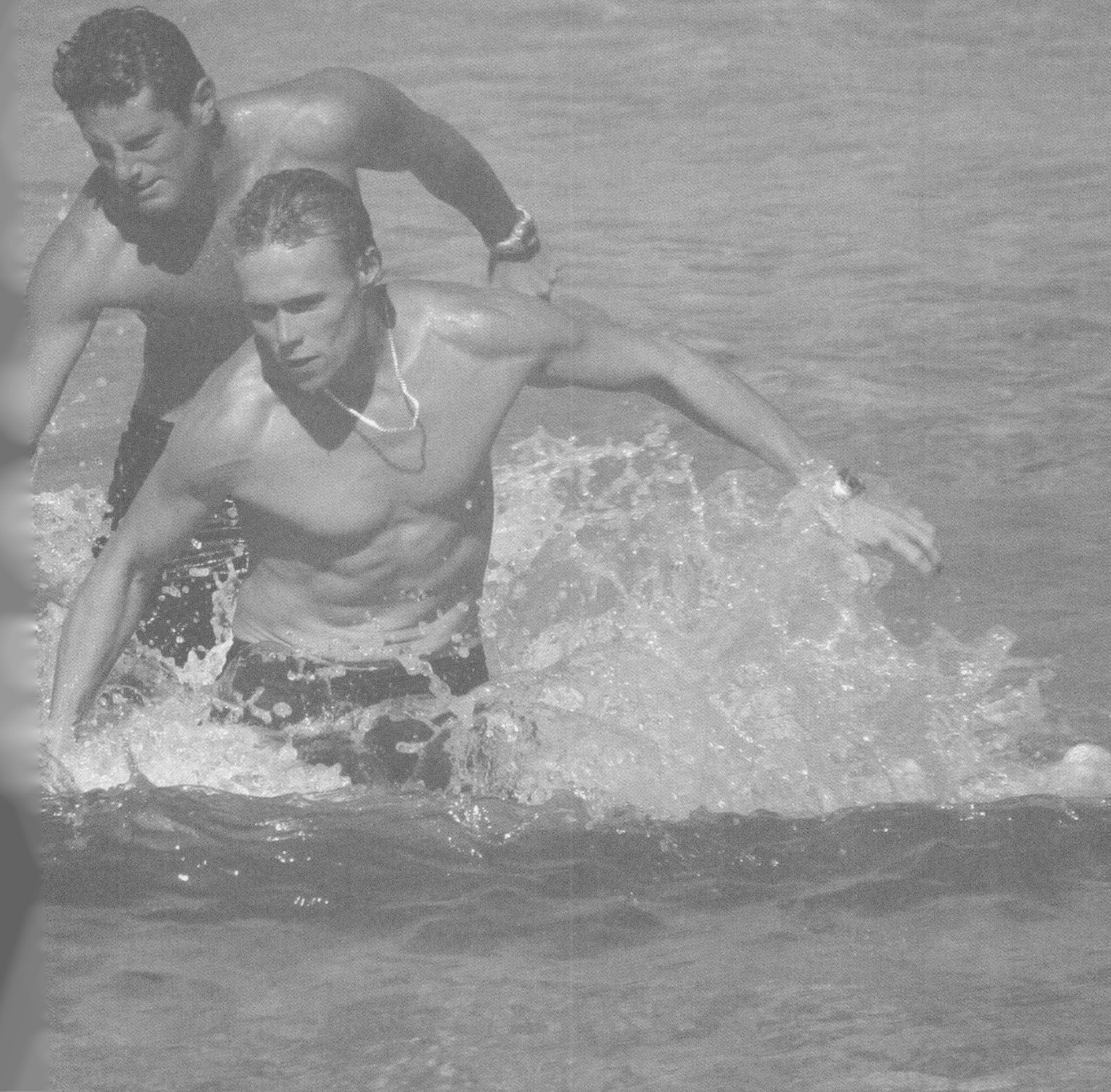

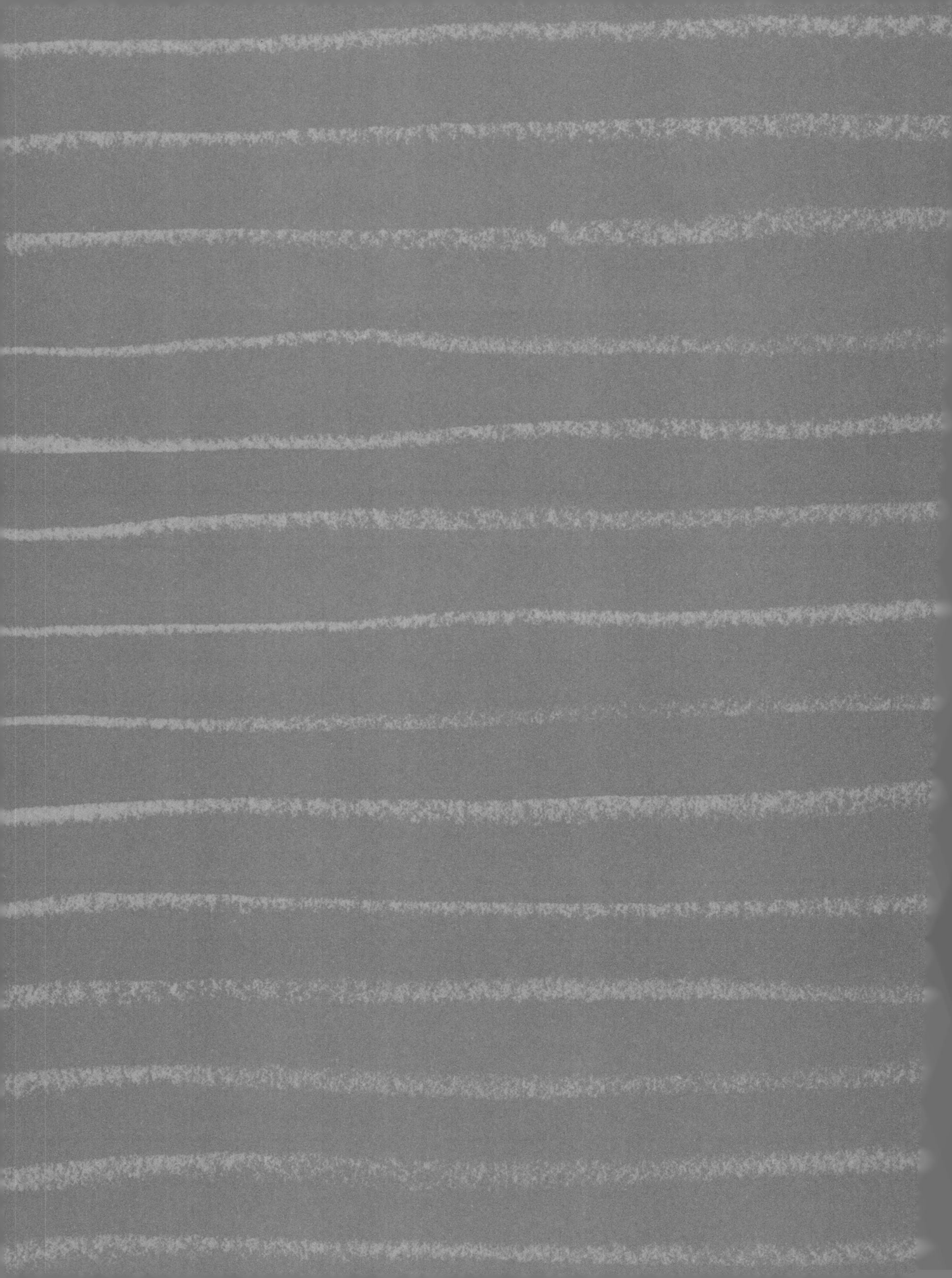

What's it like on the other end of the board?

Thousands of people have been pulled out of trouble by the Bondi lifeguard crew this decade. A smaller number, perhaps 40, have undergone critical resuscitation—literally have been brought back from the dead.

Not all of them are willing to talk about the experience. Those who are all have different stories to tell, though the bones of the tales are the same: odd coincidences, luck, gratitude, and the sense that these strange minutes, in which they've died and been returned, were hinges around which in some ways their lives have swung.

To tell the truth, when he was struck down by a heart attack and died on the stairwell of the Bondi Pavilion, Alan Sloper shouldn't even have been in Bondi. Which is odd, since it's where he was born and raised. Alan, 69 at the time he died, grew up right across the street from the pavilion, in Gould Street, where his father had a small carnival named 'Amuze-U' for the post-sun-and-surf beach crowds. Alan even joined the surf club for a little while. But at the age of ten, after his father sold the block of land where the carnival stood, he and his family moved away. Alan stuck with the family business, eventually moving his carnival's base out to Campbelltown in

Sydney's south-west basin. The Slopers wouldn't have gone to Bondi once a year.

In early 2006 Alan got a call from Waverley Council; Bondi's Festival of the Winds kite-flying weekend was on, and the council wanted the Slopers to bring out one of their carnival rides for the kids. On the day, recalls his daughter, 'We didn't really want to go. It was rainy and windy and we thought we should find out if they don't want us—then we can all have a nice day off at home.'

But no, the festival was on, no matter what, so the Slopers drove out to Bondi, set up the ride, and got to work selling tickets and snow cones and ice-cream. Alan was walking up the central stairwell of the pavilion when, he says, 'I just blacked out. Don't remember anything. Fortunately, the fellow walking behind me caught me as I went down.' That was stroke of fortune number one. Stroke of fortune number two was in the shape of the catcher, an emergency room doctor from Liverpool Hospital, who immediately began CPR while passers-by went for help.

Stroke of fortune number three came in the shape of Hoppo, who—alerted by one of the people in the pavilion—grabbed a defib unit and raced to the scene. The CPR wasn't working, but the defibrillator's shock system did. Within a couple of minutes Alan found himself back in the land of the living. Three weeks later, after specialist intervention had cleared him of any concerns, Alan returned to Bondi to say thanks to the guards who'd brought him back. He's still unable to explain why the heart attack chose that time and place to strike. 'I'd had a full check-up two weeks before and

RIGHT The fun and games stop when the oxygen mask comes out. Hoppo and Reidy at work.

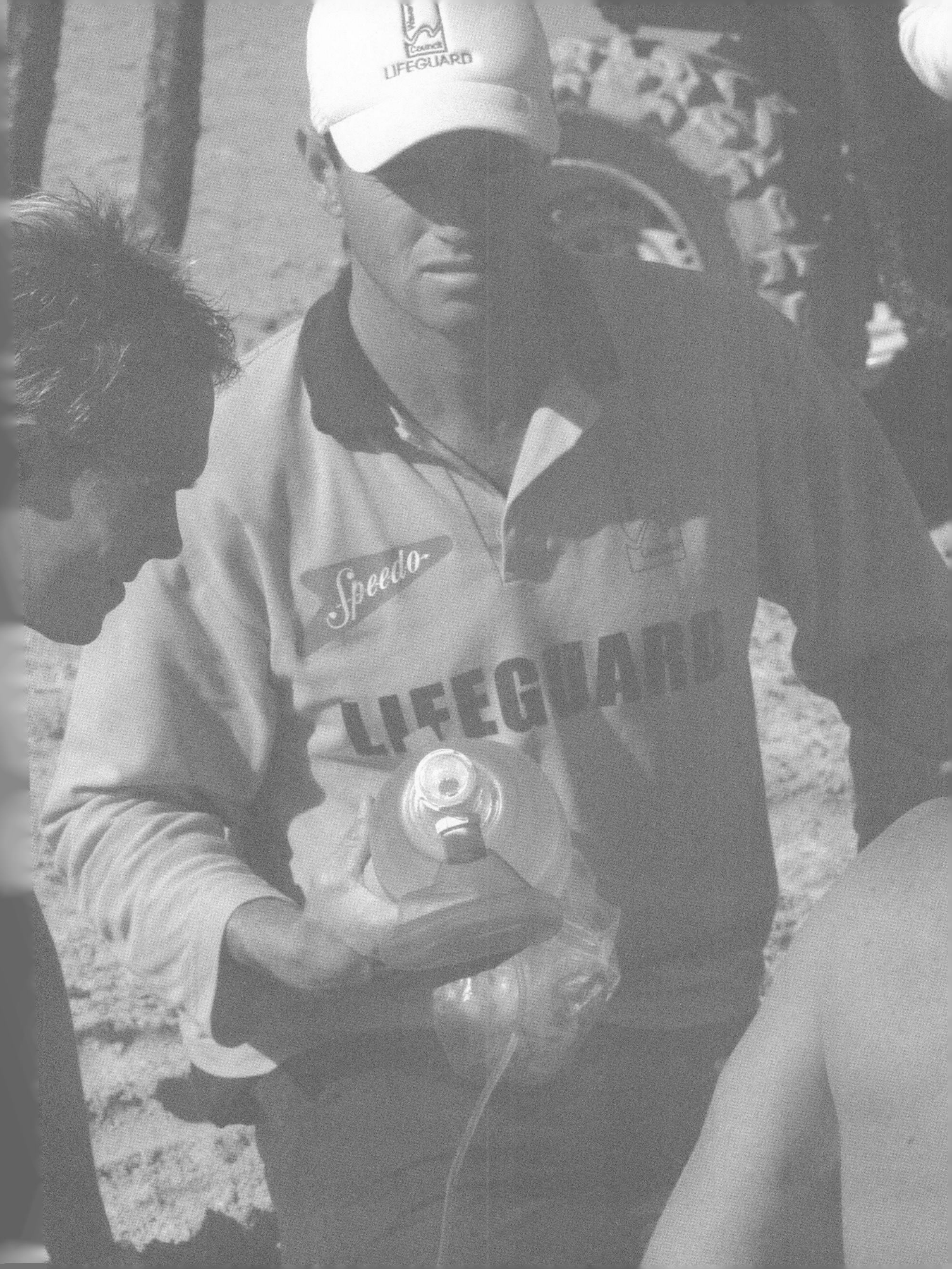
LIFEGUARD
Speedo
LIFEGUARD

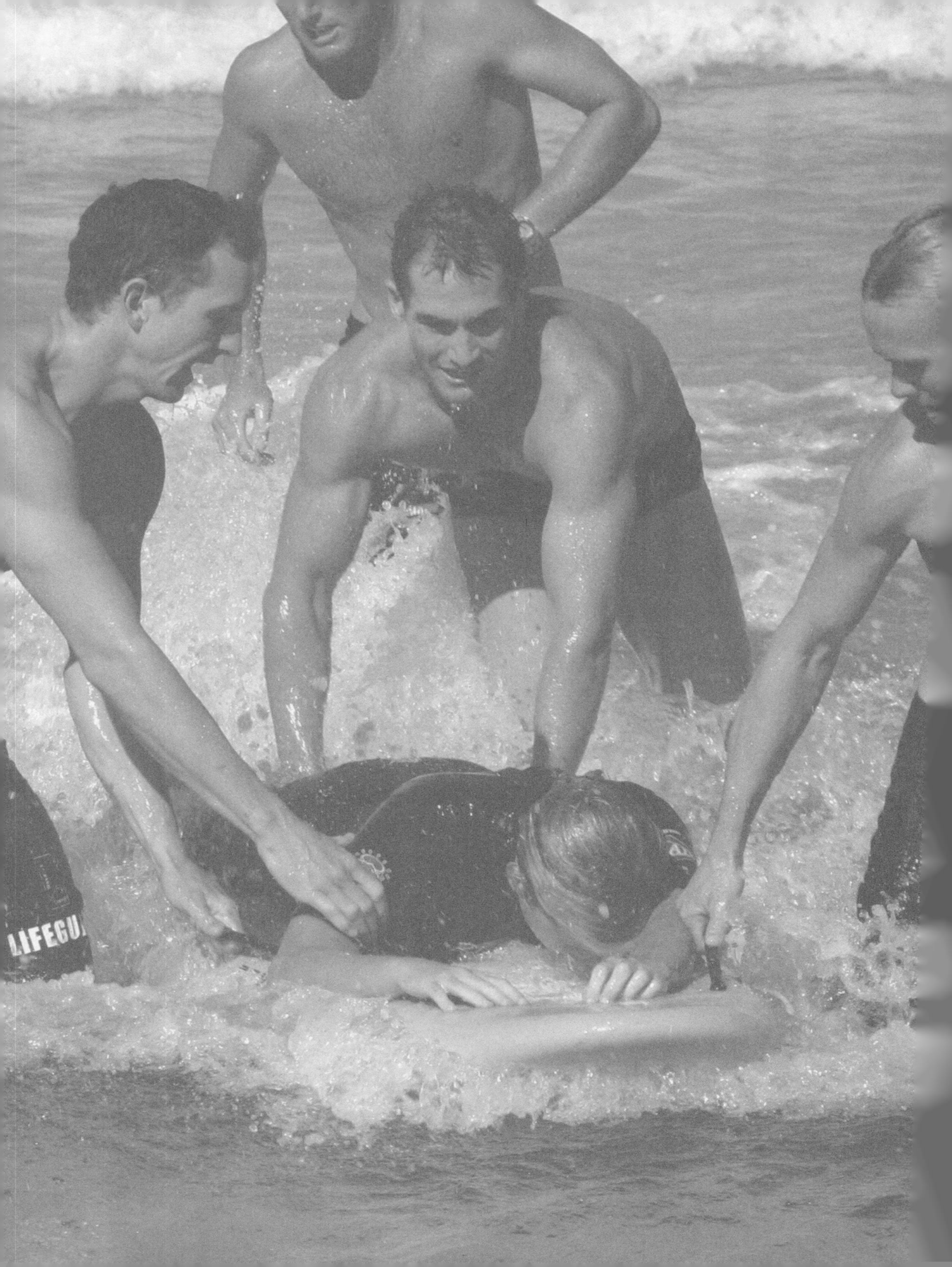
LIFEGU

there was nothing wrong,' he says. 'Afterward, the doctor did all the scans and couldn't find anything wrong either. But if I'd been anywhere else that morning, I would've stayed dead.'

Alan is 73; he and his wife recently went on a two-week *Queen Mary* cruise. 'I don't stop now,' he reckons. 'I just take it a little bit easier, that's all.'

As far as gratitude goes, Candice Tanne went to another level. She held a fundraiser on behalf of the lifeguards, three months almost to the day when she died in the surf at Bondi. Nobody really knows what happened to Candice; just that on 2 February 2005, she went surfing in heavy waves and left the water literally dead, without breath or heartbeat. Deano, Hoppo, Sean Carroll and then guard Kailin Collins were on duty at the time. Somehow they dragged her back to life and kept her going long enough for doctors to put Candice into a hypothermic coma, preventing any cascading brain damage from the oxygen starvation induced by her brief death.

Candice herself remembers only flashes of the incident. She was 26 years old at the time, a South African immigrant and a keen swimmer who'd begun learning to surf three months before. 'I've always been a water baby,' she says. 'I used to barefoot ski, I was in the swim team at school … being a sporty person helped me to get used to Australia quickly. I've always been the kind of person to throw myself into things, which probably had a lot to do with me getting into trouble that day. The surf was very rough, and it was really stupid on my part.'

She can remember locking her car, and standing on the beach getting ready to dive in, and thinking maybe she shouldn't go out.

LEFT A rescue board doubles as a stretcher in shallower water.

Then there is a brief mental flash of struggling to try to make it back to the surface. There's also a memory that's almost more of a dream—of someone putting something down her throat. (Lifeguards and paramedics have devices they use in this way to clear the airway for oxygen.) 'But it can't be a memory …' she says wonderingly. 'I had no heartbeat at the time.'

> 'Being rescued definitely gave me a lot more respect for the sea … you don't realise how quickly your life can be taken away.'

A day later she woke up in hospital, asking the same questions over and over: 'What day is it?' 'Are we at the tennis?' She thought she must still be at the Australian Open tennis tournament, where she'd been with her family a week before she drowned.

She does recall 'a sense of comfort—that you know people are around you who care about you'.

You get the sense that Candice is a strong person; the experience didn't throw her off course. 'It definitely made me reassess things,' she says. 'It didn't majorly change my personality; I'm still the same person I always was. But it has made me appreciate things more and definitely gave me a lot more respect for the sea. I used to think when I'd hear about someone drowning, "Ahh idiots, don't they know how easy it is to swim?" But you don't realise how quickly your life can be taken away.'

Four years later, her current job—Candice is a kids' swim coach who also teaches disabled kids about the water on weekends—is partly a result of her experience: 'It makes me feel like I'm doing part of my contribution to things.' She watches *Bondi Rescue* and says she loves it. 'It shows their stories and shows not to take these guys for granted. They do really care—I think you can feel that. They all took the time to talk with me and with my parents. I absolutely adore them—I owe them my life.'

Candice went swimming just four weeks after drowning, but she sold the board she'd been riding at the time, feeling it was somehow imbued with 'bad karma', and is yet to surf again. 'It's not because of what happened,' she says at first, 'it's just because of the shark thing.' But later she lets down her guard on the topic. 'There is some apprehension … I do want to go surfing again but I'm going to get Deano to come with me when I do. I think if a lifeguard is there with me, it'll help me to feel safe.'

She and her friends raised $5000 for the service. The rescue board that resulted is hanging on the wall of the lifeguard tower.

The slightly jarring thing about Tim Pearson's story is that it reinforces a blunt fact: drowning can happen to anyone. Tim is no three-month surfing rookie, and he didn't die in massive waves. He's been surfing the Bondi–Bronte area for over four decades, often in far wilder conditions than he faced in April 2009, when he paddled out one Sunday morning for a local Bondi Longboard Club surf contest heat in waves of less than a metre. A few minutes later he was being dragged back into the beach by his heat opponents with the help of a couple of alert surf club volunteers. Whippet, Dean, Reidy and Brad Malyon were among the lifeguards who got to Tim's body and shocked his heart back to work with the defibrillator. The guards were coming off the back of a dreadful Saturday when two rock fishermen had been lost off North Bondi. 'Our heads were spinning,' Dean reported. 'Local guys don't often need us that way.'

Yet sometimes they do—and when they do, like Tim, they find yet another reason to be glad they're from this beach.

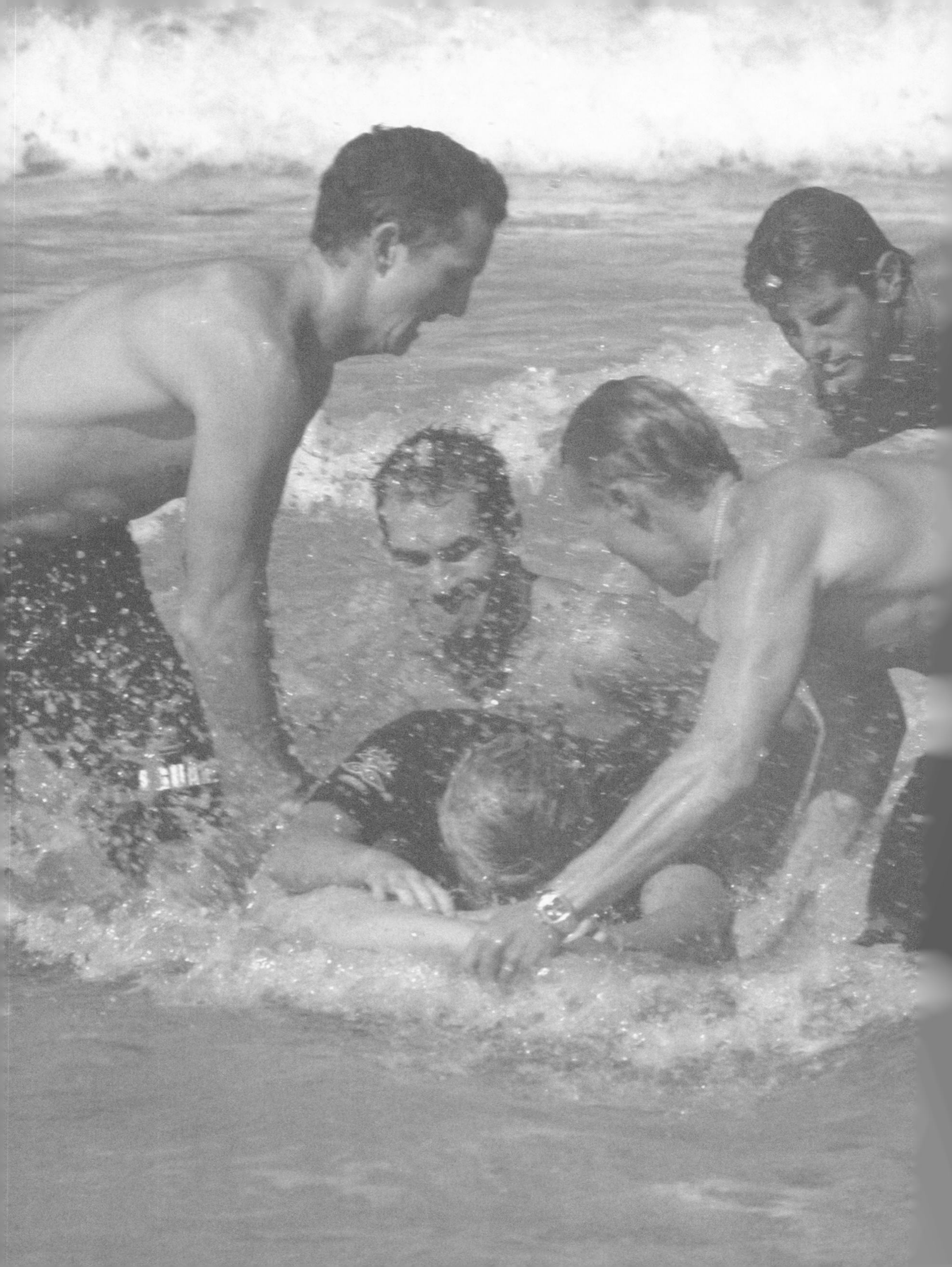

the rescued

One thing all the rescued people's stories convey—one common thread—is the lifeguards' skill and cool-headedness in a crisis. Recently a worldwide study of CPR effectiveness, mounted by the Royal Life Saving Society, returned a gloomy set of figures: on average, in all situations, CPR only works in around 5 per cent of cases. On the Waverley beaches, the rate of success is more like 95 per cent—way ahead of the curve. If you're unfortunate enough to die on a beach, just hope it's at Bondi.

LEFT Even with their experience, a rescue is always stressful–for both guards and patient.

BILL MORRIS

Corey: The Original
(Corey Oliver)

'I'd trade this off any day against working in the city. I wouldn't trade any of the money those CEOs get paid, with their headaches, not even nearly. This is where I want to lead my life, and if I can't do it through surfing or bodyboarding, I'll do it through this.'

Corey Oliver is acutely aware of his good fortune, and of how different it might've been. His parents, Raymond and Sandy, grew up in Fairfield in western Sydney, out of range of anything but weekend expeditions to the beaches he now calls home. They could easily have stayed.

As it is, though, here's Corey, feet up, deceptively relaxed in the Tamarama lifeguard tower, eyes roving across the sheltered sands of Bondi's next-door neighbour. Because Raymond and Sandy didn't stay. They moved to Clovelly when their younger son was still a toddler, and, he says, 'I thank them every day ... If it wasn't for them I wouldn't be surfing, bodyboarding, lifeguarding, everything I'm doing now. Look at the office, you know, it's really good.'

Corey's a bit of a gypsy. He lives in the Bronte surf club, the ultimate in beachside lifestyle accommodation, thanks to his off-duty job as the caretaker, and travels as much as he can; during the 2009 shark attack, for instance, he was halfway through three weeks in Switzerland. He has a piece of land down on the NSW south coast, has plans to go down there a lot more in the future, doesn't drink much or take drugs, and has very deep-set dark green eyes, a sign of his Italian heritage.

On the one hand he's a simple Aussie bloke; Whippet says 'all German backpackers should avoid Corey where possible'. But on the other he's an intelligent, clean-living person who keeps a fair bit tucked away inside. A bit of a loner, perhaps. Hidden depths. But like almost all the lifeguards, he's straight up, not given to bullshit.

He's also a *Bondi Rescue* original, who's seen the service evolve under the camera's eye. 'I think everyone has smartened themselves up a bit to be more professional and aware of what they're doing and how they're doing it. Because they know they're gonna be scrutinised on it. Personally I like it, I think it's good for the nation, it's good for the lifeguarding service, it's made our job a lot easier, it's nice to know people are paying more attention to what we do.'

Corey David Oliver was born on 16 October 1976, in Waverley War Memorial hospital. Corey's parents divorced, but not before they'd had him and older brother Shane. The two have a younger half-brother courtesy of their dad's second go-round. 'A tribe of boys,' reckons Corey. 'None of us look the same.' They saw a fair bit less of their dad after the split, once every two weeks, but Corey says, 'He's always made an effort to spend time with us.'

Raymond, a butcher, moved on to work at the security company, Brambles, where coincidentally Hoppo's dad also worked. Mum came from an adoptive background; her adopted maiden name was Hawkins, her true family name Prescott. When the laws were recently changed on adoptee information access, she found her own mum,

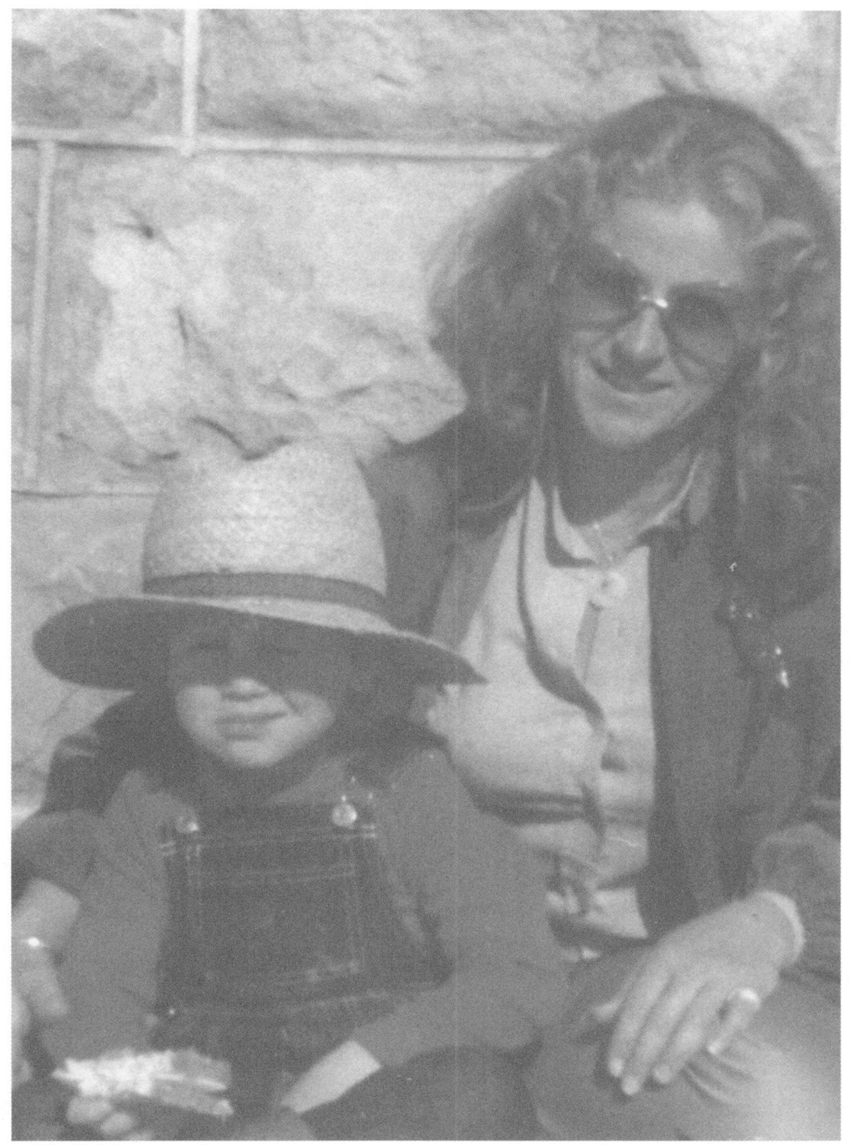

ABOVE Corey with Mum Sandy:
'she always tried to put us into swim school'.

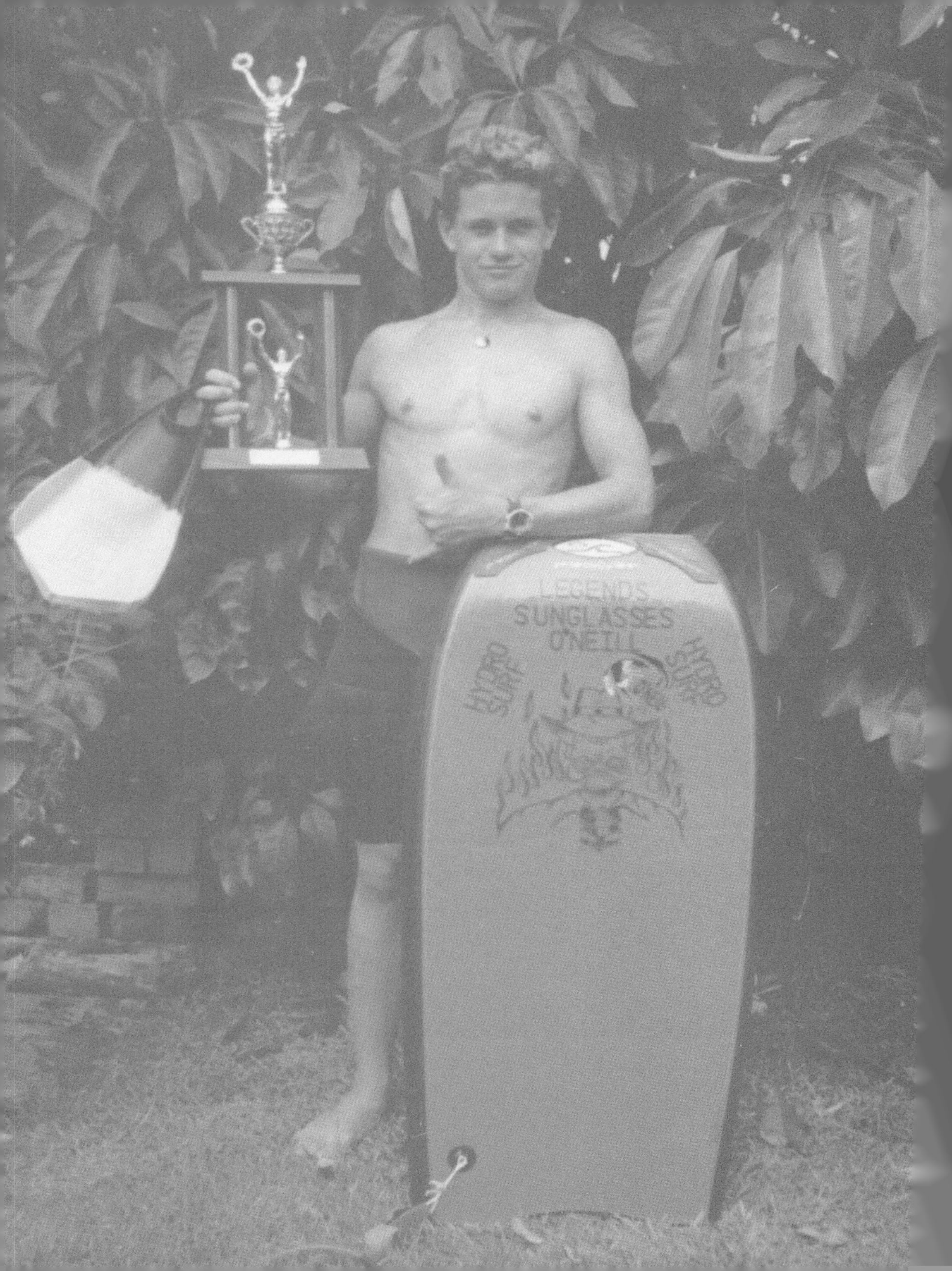
LEGENDS
SUNGLASSES
O'NEILL
HYDRO SURF
HYDRO SURF

who'd fallen pregnant by an Italian gentleman she described as 'the love of my life.' They were forced apart by the prejudices of the time, yet when Corey first met his nan, she broke down: 'She said I looked exactly the same as her Italian bloke.'

He attended Clovelly Public School and Randwick North High School, where he did design technology—his marketing task was making a bodyboard—loved art and woodwork, disliked maths, and never went to uni, partly because the surf got in the way.

Corey reckons he and Shane must've driven their mum mad. Perhaps that's why she got them outdoors whenever she could. The Oliver boys were beach kids as soon as practically possible. They did Nippers at Bronte, where Shane was a competitive swimmer. 'Mum always tried to put us into swim school. I remember we went to a swim school in Bronte pool. I wasn't strong enough to do proper freestyle, so the lady grabbed my head and dunked me underwater. Scared the absolute Christ outta me. Instilled a fear of water in me for a long time. I'd never go in swim carnivals at school and all that. My brother was a good swimmer, my mum was a great butterfly swimmer, and I hated it. Just because of that fear from that lady.'

Despite the scary initiation, or maybe in response to it, Corey got into surfing. He had an old board he didn't like—it had a loose piece of fibreglass that kept kicking up and cutting his foot—so he tossed it and began bodyboarding instead. 'I started doing competitions, I didn't really know anyone else who was bodyboarding, and I surprised myself by doing OK in some of the events.'

LEFT Corey the winner—he surprised himself with his bodyboarding success.

It was a while before he felt the culture-clash rising between bodyboarders and surfboard riders. 'All my brother's mates were surfers. We were away one weekend and Shane was allowed to stay home. Our bedrooms were covered in photos, he had [surfer] Gary Elkerton all down one wall, and I had every one of my favourite bodyboarders. We came home and every eyehole in the pictures in my room had been burned out. The boys had ripped 'em and burned 'em out. Years of gathering posters and pictures down the drain. I was devastated, ready to kill!

'But it's made me grow up with surfers and bodyboarders and get over the difference. In a way it's made me want to ride a body-board like a surfboard.'

Corey competed from the age of fourteen, just doing the Australian events, but his gypsy spirit got the better of him. He went to Hawaii, stayed there six weeks and loved the place, returning the next year, when he just missed the quarter finals at the legendary Pipeline. It was fun but hardly lucrative; he was ranked fourth in the opens in Australia when he quit, but the most he ever won in a single event was $350. 'I guess I always had the idea that I wanted to be a pro bodyboarder,' he says. 'But I think I'd had enough. I thought, "I can go up and down the coast for half the amount of money and get way better waves with two or three people".'

At the age of 20, he had to think about a real life. After some casual work at Randwick racecourse and in various surf shops, he met a bloke named Andrew Mitchell, a former soldier, who became a big inspiration. 'He was of an age that he coulda been my dad, but him and his girlfriend had never had kids, so it was kind of a bit of a link between us.' Sadly, Andrew died a couple of years ago.

Somewhere in there Corey worked at Bronte Inn above the beach, found himself down at the beach during the day, and one of

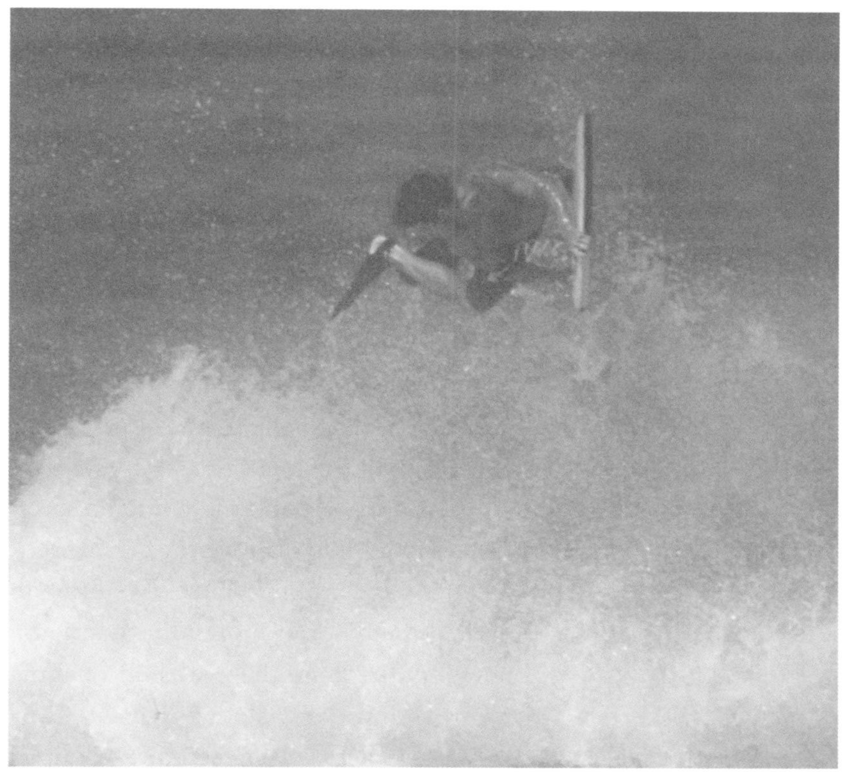

ABOVE Boom! A long way out and checking his landing site.

the lifeguards suggested he try out. He went away and got the qualifications, but Waverley only had a very casual position available, so Corey worked for Randwick Council at Maroubra, where he put in six years and 'saw some pretty fuckin' interesting things, which was an eye-opener. I thoroughly enjoyed it.'

His first-ever critical resuscitation was at Maroubra with Mark Scott, a renowned surfer/lifeguard. 'This guy OD'd in the toilets, walked out and hit the deck. We ran out with the oxygen, and thank God, he'd only stopped breathing, his heart was still beating, so we just had to breathe him up. The ambulance guys were a while, which was odd seeing as how there's an ambulance station right across the road. They gave him a shot of Narcane and within a few seconds he sat up as if nothing had happened. I was totally amazed, this guy was dead, and then he sat up. He was a bit dazed, but the ambulance guys just turned away, they'd seen things like it before. He started walking away and I was following him, waiting for him to fall over, and they're just going, "Don't worry about him, he's fine".'

'Everything I've done in my life has come from the beach. It's an Australian way of living.'

After a lifeguard conference in Grajagan in Indonesia, Corey took a break to attend big brother Shane's wedding in Ireland, and when he finally returned a few months later, there was an opening in Waverley. Corey slotted right in.

He's very clear about the social differences between the three beaches; in many ways, they're more than headlands apart. 'Bondi's definitely a lot busier. There's a lot more beach space so there's a lot more rips and a lot more very strong multicultural backgrounds, some for the better, some for the worse, unfortunately.' Bronte and Tamarama, on the other hand, occupy the same bay, with limited sand frontage and limited surf access; you can stop bad things happening a bit more easily than at the super-crowded, wide open Bondi.

Tamarama, where he's working today, is like a little amphitheatre. There's only one shop and minimal parking. People come there to escape the crowds at all the other beaches. 'It's not as busy,' Corey says, 'but when the shit hits the fan it's really tricky.'

Examples leap to mind. Once he had to pull in a guy who'd slipped off the Tama cliffs. The guy was from Melbourne, had been walking around the cliff top, and thought he'd climb over the walkway fence and take some photos. 'We were surfing at Mackenzie's and all of a sudden the whole walkway started screaming. I'd seen what was going on and this other surfer came with me, turns out he'd been a lifeguard in Western Australia at some point so he was able to help me. We got there and the guy was torn to pieces from rolling on the rocks, a massive hole in his head. We got the bodyboard under him, then the surfboard too, so he had some support. The other guy put a couple of breaths into him but I was totally amazed that he did, the hole in his head was like a 50-cent coin and it was right through, a horrific sight. He was foaming and his body started reacting and convulsing.' A couple of the Bondi guards came round on a jet ski and they all brought him in to Tamarama. The ambulance was already there and ready. 'To see the ambulance here was unreal. But even the ambulance guys went, "Oh, no way." Everyone's gonna see something like that, and if you can't stand it, you shouldn't do it ... it'll screw with your head.'

Corey is very intense on the subject of coping with the extremes encountered in his job. On another day at Bondi some time later, he explains the difficult things: the families of suicides, the body retrievals, the knowledge that sometimes you can't do anything but protect the dignity of the dead, even if it means taking them out to sea to wait for a beach crowd to be cleared. 'I like to be there for that stuff, because I know I'll give the person every bit of dignity I can. That's one way I can feel better about it.'

Meanwhile, between the peak moments, there's days like today at Tamarama—light winds, small waves, time to enjoy the job. An American girl comes up to the tower, looking for some sunscreen to protect a freshly minted tattoo across the elegant small of her back; Corey applies it with a slight grin.

How long can this last? 'I'd love to see myself going through time. [Lifeguard] Harry Nightingale is nearly 60, I think. He's pretty fit, he's a great swimmer, he's always going to Indonesia, I think he's had a second wind in his life.'

Corey has the idea that when it comes to settling down and having a family, he'll do it at the beach, the way his parents did for him. 'Everything I've done has come from the beach. It's an Australian way of living.'

RIGHT Not the worst life you can imagine. Corey takes a lunch break at the south end.

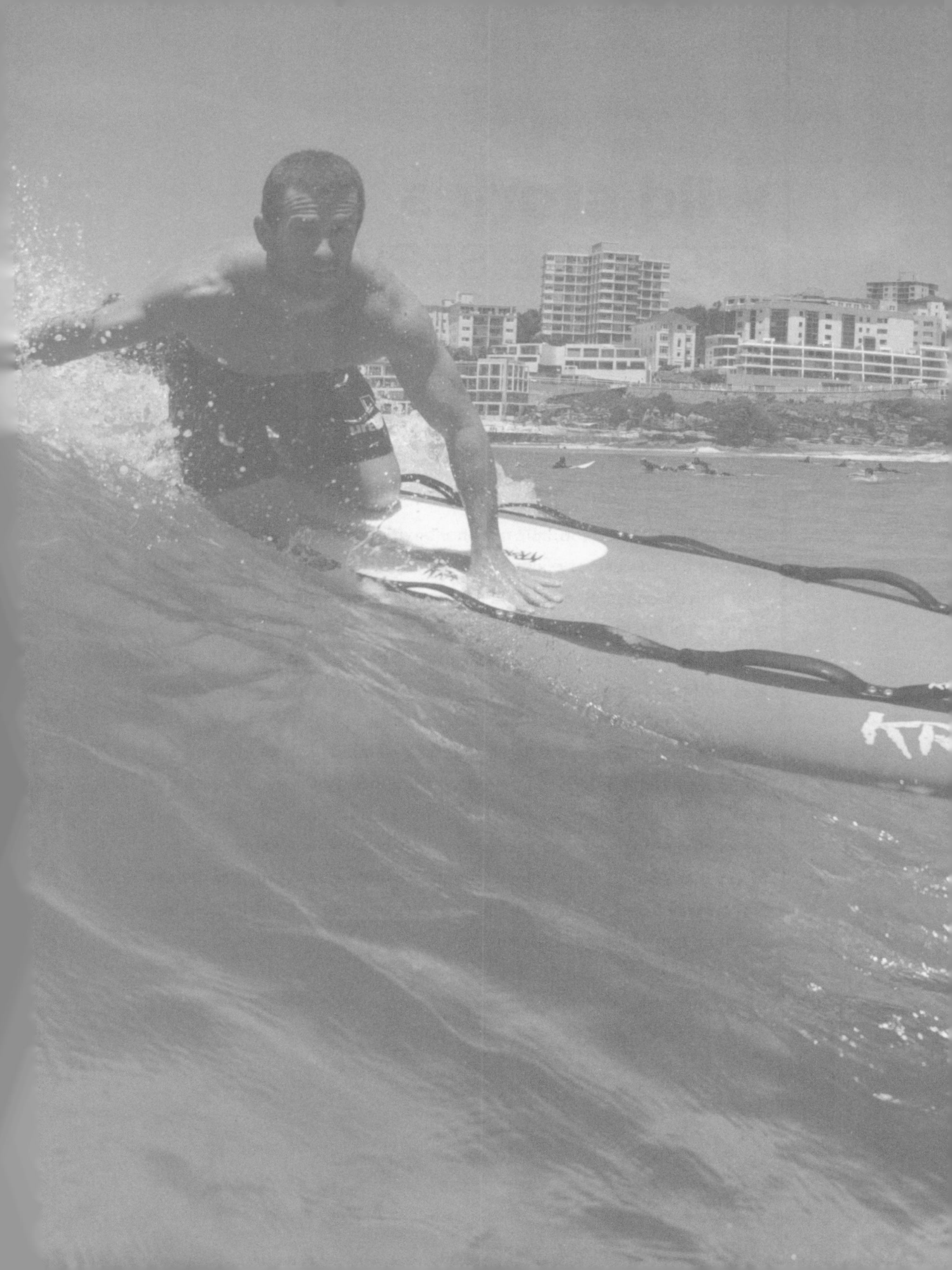

wild stories FROM THE SERVICE

The girl who jumped

SHE'D LOST HER job, split from her boyfriend, and, on top of it, learned she had a mild case of epilepsy—just enough to prevent her from safely travelling overseas. She couldn't see past it, so on a morning in late 2007, she went alone to the cliffs of south Bondi, and jumped.

Hoppo and Corey took the call and retrieved her on the jet ski. There was nothing they could do other than secure her remains ... and later, open themselves to a visit from her parents.

Something about this girl and the subsequent visit has stayed with the crew, almost as if it happened yesterday. Says Corey: 'I don't know what's harder, dealing with the situation and looking after the patient respectfully—cos everyone gawks—or whether it's when the parents come to say thank you. It was so confronting. The mum was crying and the dad was heavily upset, she'd been the apple of their eye. It's hard to see how much of an effect it has on a family.'

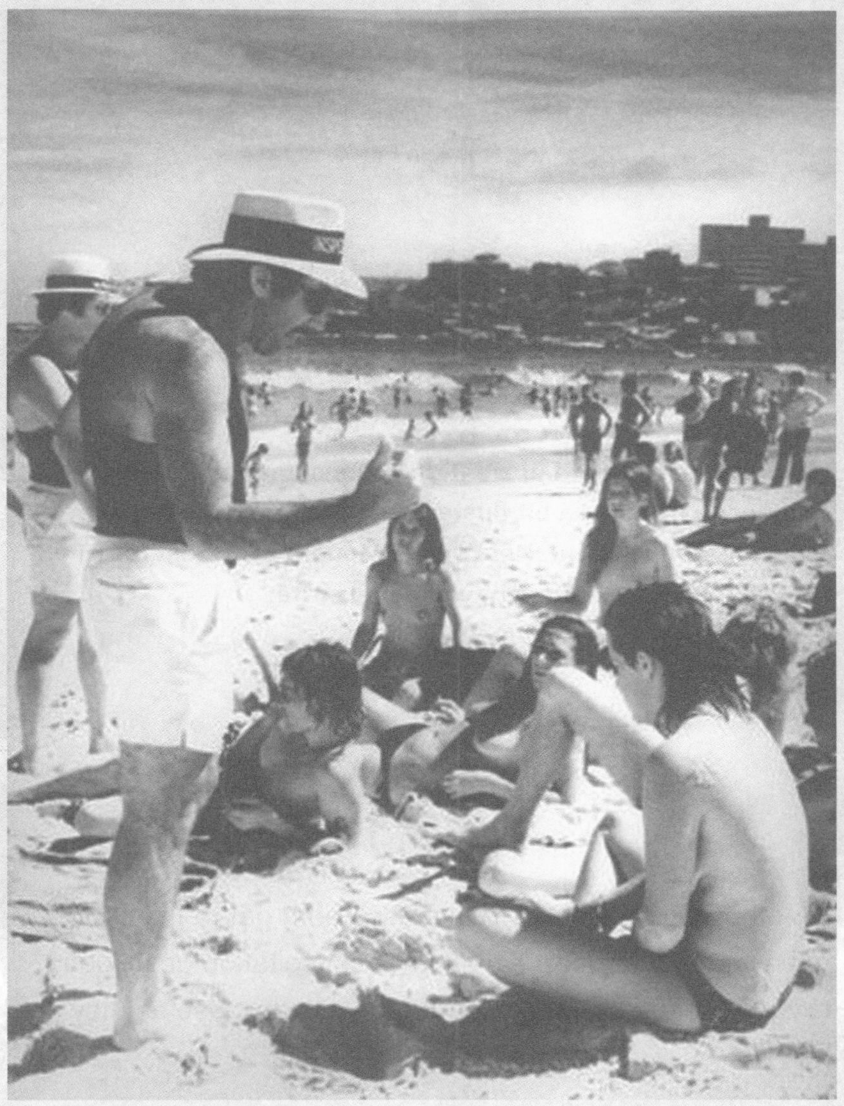

ABOVE Busted! 1972, and Beach Inspector Allen Johnston performs the first topless bathing arrests in Bondi history. Those were the days.

TOP 8 Critical rescue actions

There's the standard prevention actions, then there's bringing someone in who's a bit flustered–then there's the big one, an unconscious patient. Here's the lifeguard check-list for when someone's in real strife:

1. Mobilise

'Get there,' says Deano. This means both get to the patient in the water, and get the high-end resuscitation gear–defib, oxygen–set up and ready on the beach, as close as they can get to the point of exit.

2. Call for assistance

The rescuer has a special signal—one fist pumped up and down three times—to indicate an unconscious patient; this lets the beach crew know what they're in for, and prompts an immediate 000 call for ambulance backup.

3. Get the victim to the beach ASAP

'Some manuals say to get a couple of breaths into 'em while you're out there,' says Hoppo, 'but realistically, it's a bit of a waste of time ... We can do way more for 'em on the sand.'

4. Performing CPR

Use the Oxy-Viva oxygen-delivery system and external heart massage with the defibrillator monitoring their progress. The lifeguards will continue this, revolving the duties (heart massage is a strenuous effort), until the patient regains consciousness or until they're relieved by paramedics.

5. Stabilise the patient

Someone re-emerging into consciousness may go into shock; he or she may have other injuries. In any case, the patient will need close monitoring and further oxygen therapy, and the lifeguards will work with him/her to get as much information as they can about the patient's state, family contacts etc.

6. Clean up

Things left at the rescue scene can leave quite a trail. Glenn Orgias, the January shark attack victim, had left his car key in his surfboard's leg-rope pocket; Glenn's brother had no idea how to move the car, until the leg-rope was found back at the tower.

7. Debrief/report

Every critical rescue/resuscitation is talked through and analysed; important information may or may not come up straightaway, but each debrief adds to the lifeguards' understanding of what leads up to these potentially lethal events.

8. Counselling

This is increasingly being recognised as a necessary step, says Hoppo. 'In the old days, you'd just get on with it,' he reckons. 'But a young lifeguard, confronted with a suicide for instance, that's a traumatic event, and it might not surface for months.'

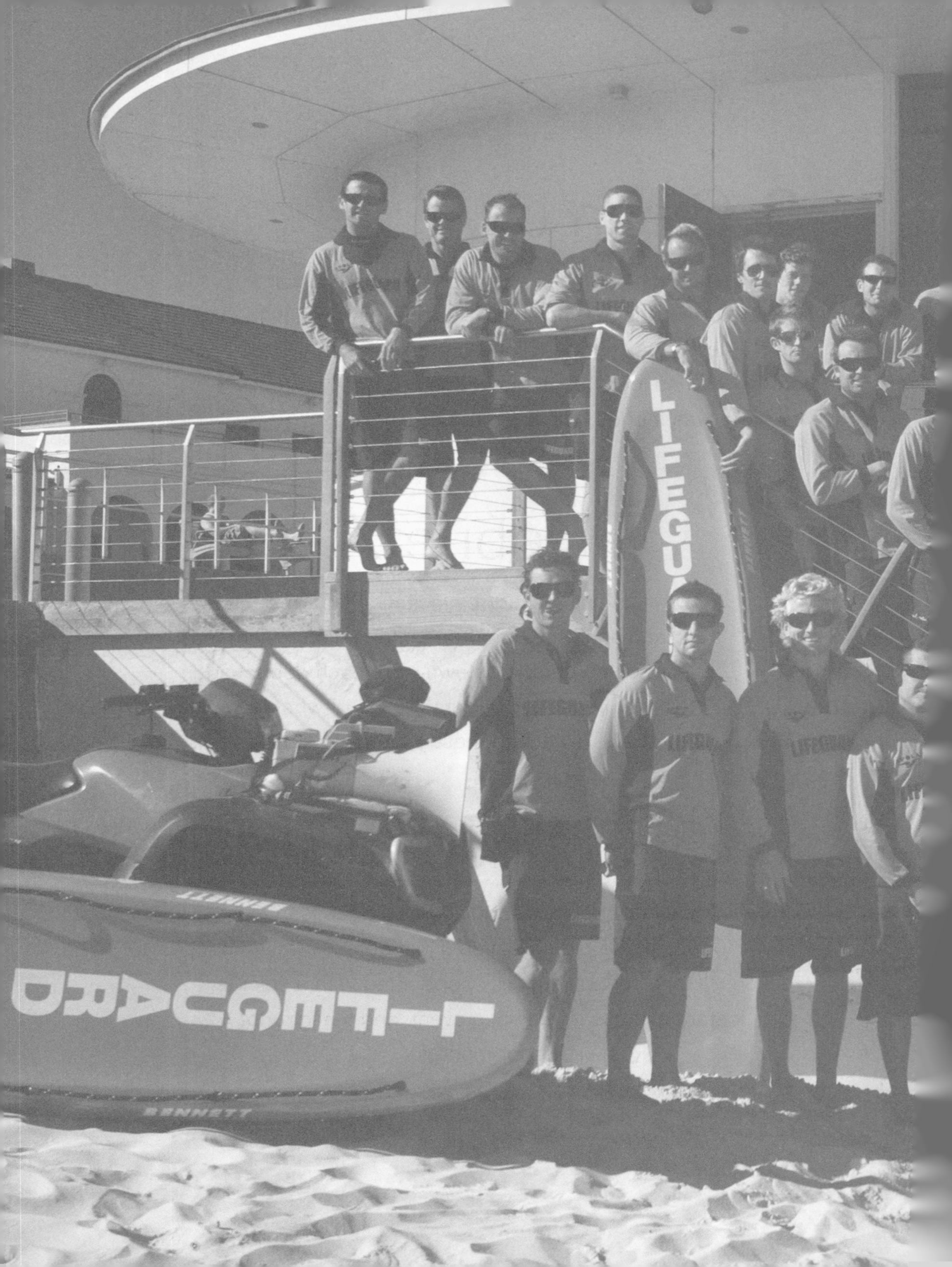
LIFEGUA
BENNETT

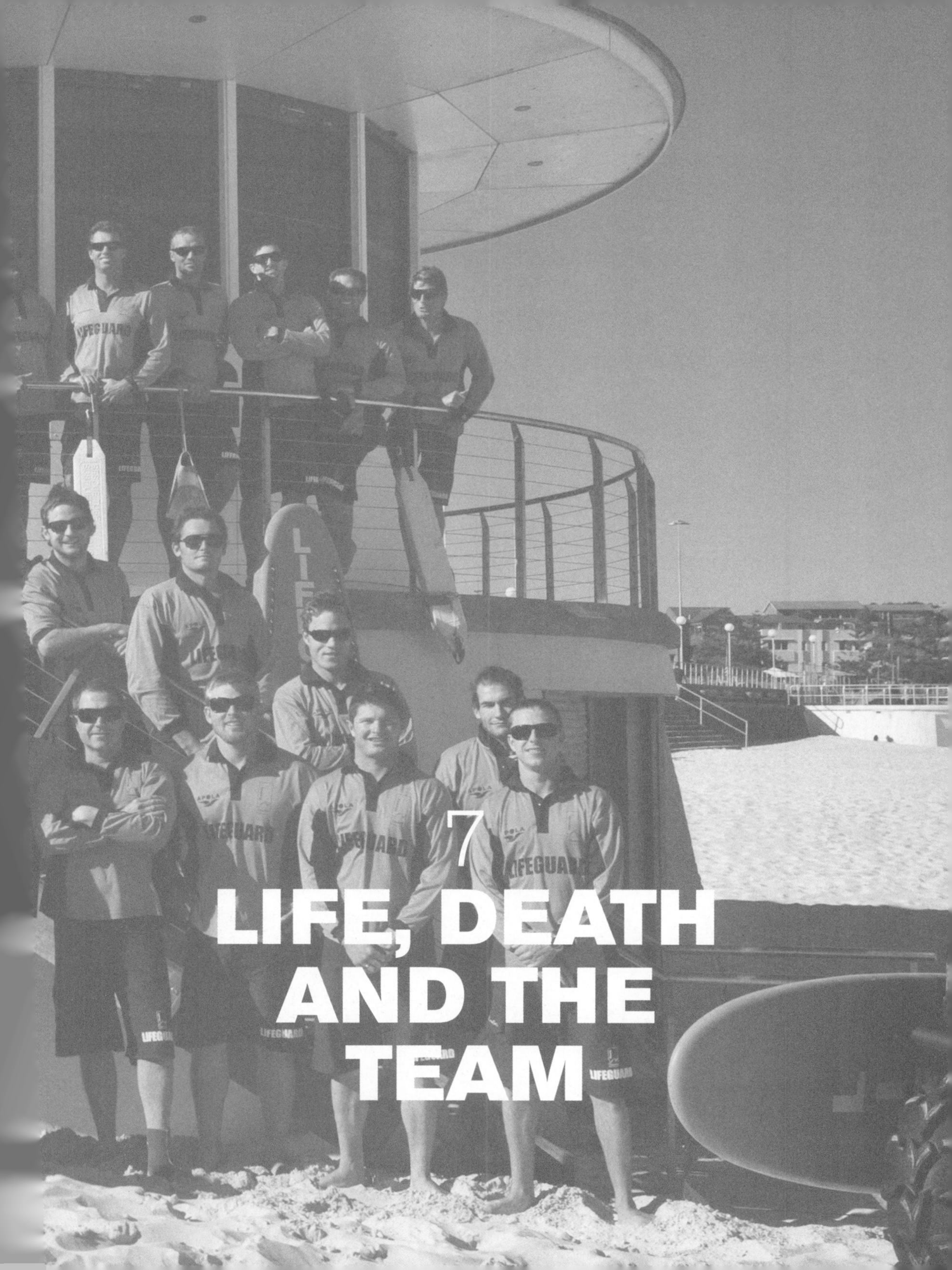

7 LIFE, DEATH AND THE TEAM

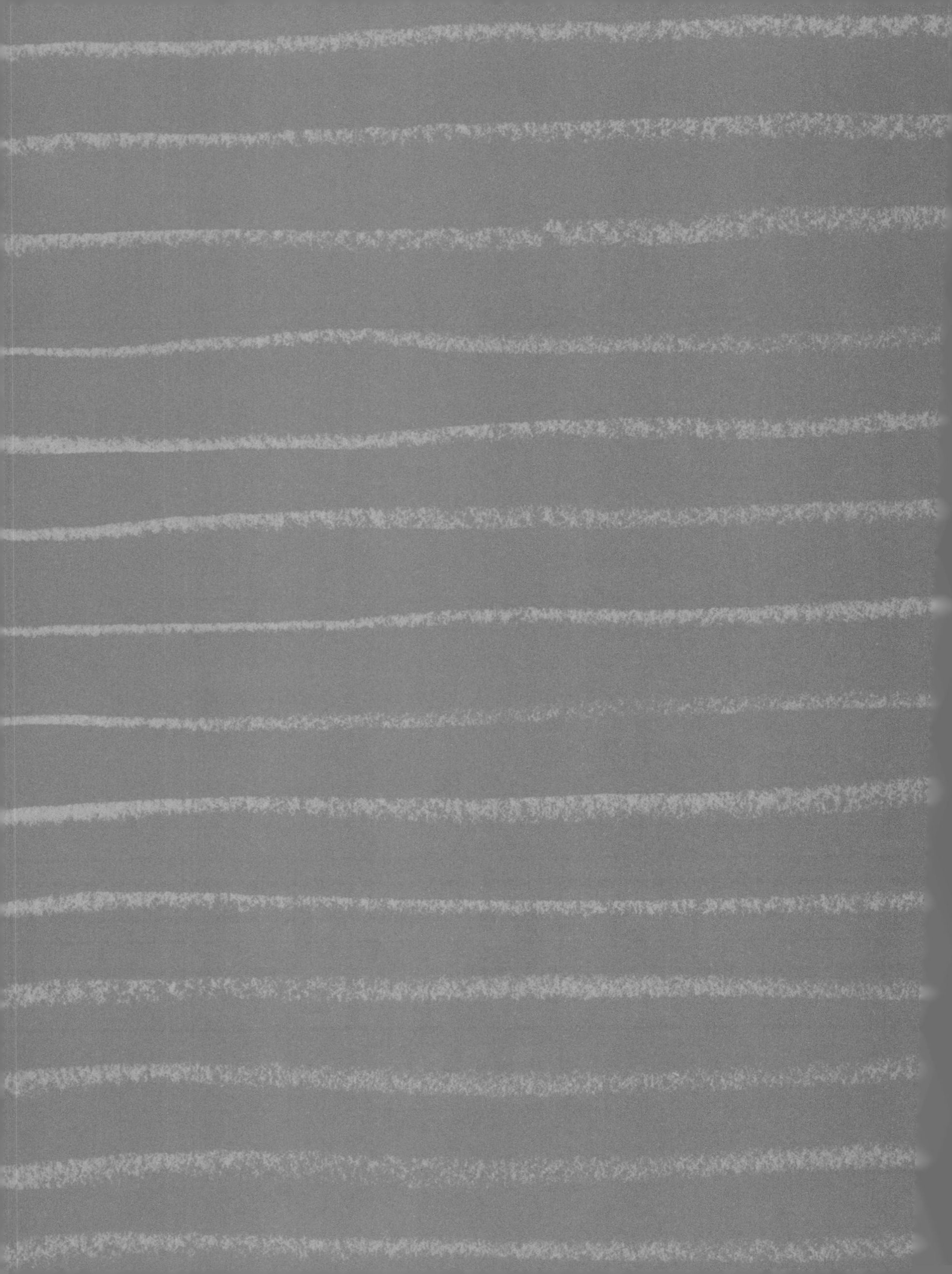

They don't just look after you, but after each other too

Here's a little home truth about lifeguarding: risky rescues are actually fun. They're an adrenaline rush.

'It is entertaining for us for sure,' says Harries, shaking his head over some of his clients. 'They've got no idea. Half of 'em, their cossies fall off ... I mean the hardest thing for a girl, you tell 'em to open their legs so you can lie them on the board, you say, "Well, what do you want? You want to open your legs so I can get you back to shore, or you want to drown?" You end up saying, "Listen darlin', I've seen thousands of 'em." You don't want to put a lady in a bad situation, but ... sometimes you just gotta just spread 'em!'

The Bondi lifeguards are a lot of things: comedians, surf addicts, students, girl-chasers, pros, even the occasional grown-up. But at work, above all, they're a team. All their stories, all their efforts and training and memories and easygoing jokes and pranks, come back to this—the need to unquestioningly rely on one another.

This team bond revolves around another, far more potent home truth, one they rarely discuss yet live with every working day: The lifeguards know their job will regularly bring them into direct contact with the death of a fellow human being.

Waterborne emergencies happen swiftly, sometimes rather mysteriously. You can be watching someone near a rip, switch your attention somewhere else for a few seconds, and turn back and the person is gone, or in deep difficulties ... and people in the water become LESS visible when in trouble, not more visible the way they would on land. They go down, below the waterline. They're in over their heads.

And in a way, when they go under, they're taking the lifeguards with them—into deeper water than most people are forced to stray.

You hear it in the boys' descriptions: The 'Ring of Death', describing how people tend to gather around an unconscious patient on a beach. You hear it in their horror of working 'one-out', the way Hoppo had to do in his first few years, left alone in charge of a crowded beach.

You hear it in the way they describe the part of a lifeguard's job that seems almost magical—the resuscitation of a person who is by most judgements already dead. The stories almost always peak with six or seven guards, having responded to the call of their teammate, working together in near-silence but for the radio and the robotic voice of the defibrillator, re-creating the rhythm of the victim's heartbeat and breath, all aware it could tip either way. 'It's an amazing feeling, to actually see someone die in your arms,' says Harries, recounting his part in the freakish rescue of two drowning victims in Bali in 2008. 'Death doesn't bother me at all. I shouldn't say it, I really enjoy the training, I've been involved with so many critical situations that it doesn't bother me cos I get so much out of it. It's a learning curve for me. In Bali, this guy was dying in my arms. One of the lifeguards was running around on the ATV we'd donated to 'em the day before. So I've picked him up like he was a 5-kilo weight, threw him over me and we were driving around the back streets of Kuta with a dead person in my arms. He looked like a puppet.' Amazingly, they managed to save the man.

Harries says, 'It's a great feeling to know that you've seen 'em on their way to heaven and then bring 'em back maybe to heaven on earth. I feel blessed to have been able to do that for someone.'

If successful resuscitation is the best feeling in lifeguarding, suicide recovery is the worst. Hoppo describes a 'dead smell' on the hands after you've handled a body, some exhalation from the skin that can't be washed off for some time. He remembers a man who used to ride down to the tower on a motorbike every day and yell out about how the guards had the best job in the world and how lucky they were. Then one morning Hoppo had to retrieve a 25-year-old girl who'd jumped off the cliff at the south end. She'd hit something on the way down and it'd sheared half her head away. Later when the guy rode down on his motorbike, Hoppo explained what had happened that morning; the guy shut up and never did it again.

The families of suicides often need to talk with the lifeguards involved, which they understand, yet that takes its own particular kind of toll. 'None of us have training for that,' says Hoppo.

Not everybody makes it past the moments of truth. Occasionally a guard will suffer a kind of post-traumatic stress breakdown. One guy a few years ago had to deal with two dead bodies in a week; during the second retrieval, while waiting with the body for a helicopter pickup, he'd kept the body afloat by fitting it with a rescue tube. When the helicopter rescue swimmer came down and put a pickup harness on the body, the tube was accidentally caught underneath it, with the result that the lifeguard was hauled out of the water together with the body, attached by the rescue tube line to his own harness.

Hoppo remembers him fighting in a panic to get out of the harness, and finally freeing himself and falling back into the water.

Something about the incident just pushed the lifeguard over the limit. 'He wasn't the same after that,' Hoppo says. 'He didn't come back next season.'

Another guard, in trying to rescue a swimmer along the Tamarama cliff line, was washed into a cave and pinned. Eventually he fought free, but again, was never quite the same afterward.

Those who get past the moments of truth evolve some interesting philosophies. Corey Oliver's had a range of nicknames levelled at him through the past year, notably the 'Bone Collector'. This one stemmed from his presence at both Waverley's beach suicides and one of its critical resuscitations for 2009. He says the events haven't unduly bothered him. Corey says he believes in memory—that a person lives on through the memories engendered in the minds of family and friends. Like the other lifeguards, he finds it hard when a victim's family comes to meet him; it erases the pretension of distance and makes the event real, concrete.

Harries, on the other hand, sounds like he's the service's first homegrown existentialist. 'To see someone die is a really traumatic thing. I feel more for the family than for myself, cos I know if I do a really good job to try to get this kid back to their family, they won't mourn as much. They might be going to a better place or it might just be their time. But it does affect me when I meet their families, cos they will be really humble—they'll come up and say, "I just want you to know how much we appreciated your help, my son was in so much pain from depression and you tried everything you could." And to hear that is just amazing. You give the mother a cuddle, and a mother is so close to her child. That's probably the only time I feel a bit of emotion and get a bit throaty. This is a loved one. This was a walking, talking person. So I really pride myself on preserving human life. That's a good part about this job.

'But one thing I can't believe ... We're sitting here now, you and I. And we've got our ways, we get up in the morning, have a cup of coffee, then go surfing or whatever. And then—all of a sudden—you and I—WE could be dead! Just like that! In a heartbeat! It's amazing. I was out surfing once, I was doing a board training session, and I turned my head and I saw a chick land in the water. She'd committed suicide, jumped off the cliff. I sat up on the board and watched as she hit the rock, head-first. I thought, "She's DEAD. I'm alive and she's dead. I can't believe it!"'

His next-door neighbour at Clovelly, an old boozy bloke who'd won a lottery, had a saying—'Here today, gone tomorrow!' It's something that Harries has never forgotten: 'Every day you'd walk down the street ... "Here today gone tomorrow!" Life is so valuable and I feel for people who are really stressed out and suffering depression, cos life doesn't last too long, it goes so quick, just don't betray yourself for happiness.'

The lifeguards find it hard when a victim's family comes to meet them—it somehow makes the event real, concrete.

There's not much talk of religion among the lifeguard service; in a way, it's one of the most Australian things about them. Tom Bunting does still say a few prayers for the family of the Mongolian doctor who drowned on his watch in 2007—'But that doesn't mean I'm very religious,' he explains. 'I'm not dogmatic about God. But for me personally, it's important to have or take some time to acknowledge something to myself. The point is that you've taken the time to set aside to think about something else other than yourself.'

Their best defence against trauma is the knowledge that it can be shared with their peers. Much as the boys are happy with the TV series and its effect on public knowledge of their tasks, you get the feeling that they'd ditch it in a second if it proved too disruptive to the team. At times, they've all noted a risk that the show itself, with its unavoidable tendency to make stars out of some of the crew, might break down the team structure.

> 'If you want a TV career that's great but we will be here for many more rescues to come, and that's what makes us special.'

At other times, it's clear the risk is pretty slim. Close to the end of the season, after the death of a rock fisherman and the resuscitation of Tim Pearson, senior lifeguard Ben Quigley was moved to email the whole team, to acknowledge the harsh weekend and the great work done. It led to an exchange of notes between the boys that perhaps says more about the team's general mood than anything else.

This is what Harries wrote: 'I know this show has done fantastic things for all of us, but pulling up in the car park watching the boys do a resusc to a longboarder that we all know really well and defibbing him back to a living state of knowing where he was and who also brought him back to life is so good.

'If you want a TV career that's unreal but we and that's you and I will be here for many more resusc to come, and that's what makes us special. You can be a hero or a saint but don't need a audience to show your magic.

'Just over here at Bronte working hard and my eyes are on the water while I'm typing this?? But love all of you fellows for your good hearts and giving a shit at work when it matters and for a fun happy season.

'Stay positive because your thoughts become your actions and your actions become your destiny.

'PS Rodney got a modelling job with Wendy's, he has two ice cream cones on his chest.'

To which Whippet responds: 'Epic team to be a part of.

'PS. If it's not that busy this week and next weekend can we all make a big effort to help Harries with his spelling. Only a couple of new words a day will make a big difference.'

And from Corey: 'Epic job, and I am so stoked to have been on the beach this year with an awesome bunch of fun, mad, normal, interesting and positive people. I hope there are many more years of the same thing to come.

'PS. The swell will be pumping in the morning!!!! Get your froth on!'

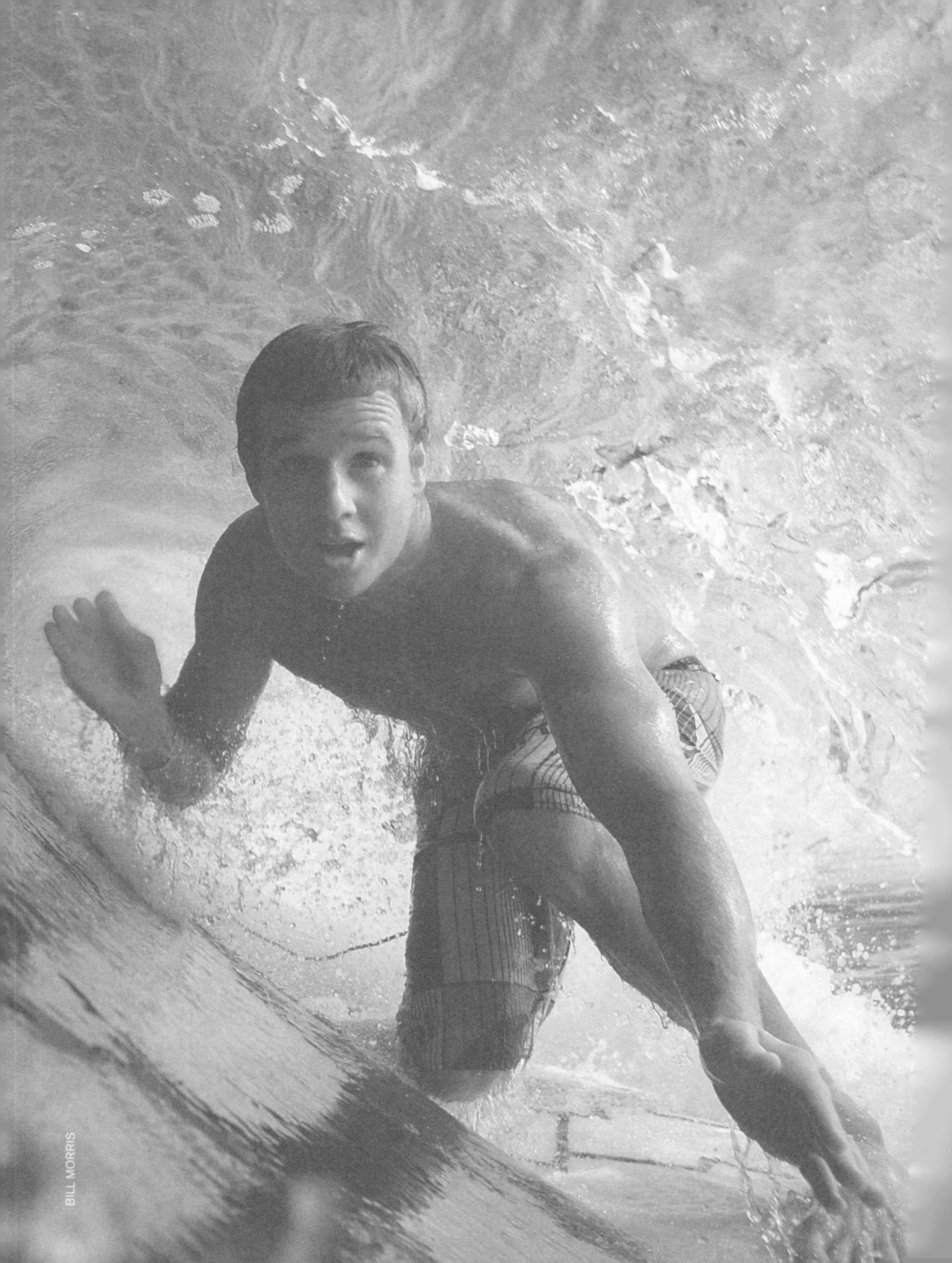

BILL MORRIS

Whippet: The Surfer
(Ryan Clark)

'There's nothing better than when there's stuff happening. When someone yells over the radio, "Get there now!" and you do, it feels like it takes ten seconds to cover that ground … Everyone's at their best when this beach is at its worst.'

Ryan 'Whippet' Clark is on a lunch break, hunched over a chicken burger at one of the pavilion's cafes, and while he's describing the sensation of embarking on a life-or-death surf rescue mission, his eyes are alight with what can only be described as surf stoke.

If the lifeguard's number-one credential is as Dean Gladstone thinks—surfing skill—then Whippet is the model of the Bondi lifeguard of today and tomorrow. He's been riding waves almost since he could walk. You also get the distinct feeling that—like a lot of lifeguards and almost all good surfers—he's a bit of a thrillseeker.

Ryan James Clark, born 9 April 1983, at Paddington Women's Hospital, is a Bronte boy through and through. His immediate family's story sounds like a microcosm of the Australian dream. His dad, Peter, is originally from Coonabarabran in western New South

Wales, where his parents had a farm and he rode a horse to school every day.

Peter Clark started surfing at the age of seventeen, when he first moved to Sydney in order to join the army and was bitten by the water bug. 'He pretty much got a panel van and did the whole east coast surfer lifestyle thing,' says Ryan. 'He's got stories from down at Bells Beach and all that.' Peter eventually settled back in Sydney and met wife Sandra, a Bondi girl; they've been married for more than 30 years. He became a builder, formed his own building company, and developed it into an insurance contractor. Sandra, Ryan's elder brother Cameron, and elder sister Alana all work there.

'I never really thought acting was something I wanted to do, I just fell into it, but I ended up loving it.'

Like Box, Ryan still lives in the same house he grew up in, with Cameron and his family (wife and two kids, seven-year-old and three-year-old girls, whom he loves), plus Ryan's girlfriend.

Sandra and Peter bought another house for themselves up the road, and live there with Lauren, at thirteen, the baby of the family.

Ryan is a casual, sleepy-eyed, friendly kid; alert, fit and very self-confident without a trace of arrogance. Of all the lifeguards, he's the one who most seems to be leading a charmed sort of life—dwelling in the bosom of a sturdy family, yet having wacky career opportunities apparently landing in his lap. For instance, he's the only one of the crew with prior experience of television; at the age of seven Ryan took a role on the beach-driven soap opera *Home and Away*. That's right, he's been a TV star twice.

whippet the surfer

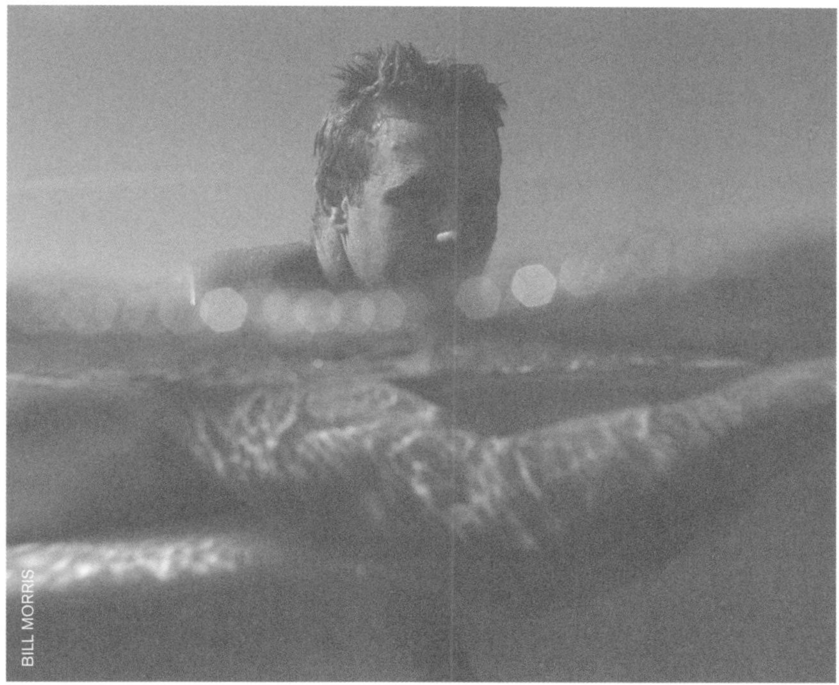

ABOVE Surfing, like acting, was something Ryan couldn't have avoided even if he'd wanted to.

How the heck do you become a television actor at the age of seven? 'A coupla family friends did a Cottee's cordial ad,' he explains, 'and Mum decided why not put the kids in an agency and see what happens? Being the little brother, I wanted to do it too, and a month later they said there's an audition for a spot, it's good practice even if you don't get it. Nine years later I was still there.

'It's a bit of a spin-out, I mean I never really thought acting was something I wanted to do, I just fell into it, but I ended up loving it.' He attended school as much as possible between shoots. Sandra

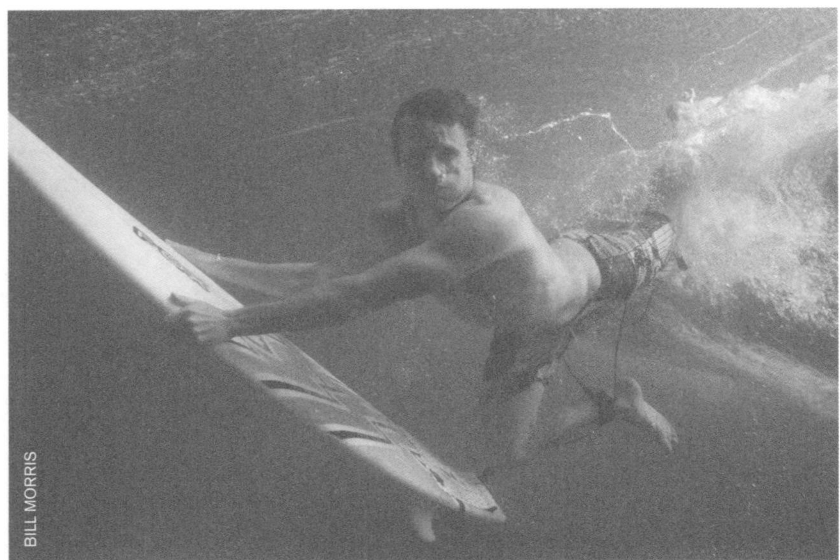

ABOVE It's another world.
Duckdiving a small one at south end.

was a teacher's aide at his high school and helped, and classmates brought him handouts.

Ryan's a very good athlete; he'd have taken out the Lifeguard Challenge in 2009 if it weren't for Harries's beach-sprinting skills. He feels competitive, which he thinks must arise from being the younger boy in a family, battling for attention with all his siblings.

Yet luckily, Cameron, five years his senior, let him tag along to all their surfing adventures. 'He got into everything before I did, so I was always the little grommet kicking around in the boot of the car, going surfing with 'em or to footy. I think my first memories would be of the Bogey Hole at Bronte, the little rockpool there, thinking I was ripping it up on a foamie.'

He remembers going surfing on longboards in Waikiki at the age of five with his dad. Did the surf club Nippers program as well: 'I didn't take it too seriously, but as a way of getting an understanding of the water it was awesome.'

'Days when it's big and there's a few guys out there surfing, if something goes wrong and I don't go get 'em, nobody else is going to.'

His nickname, Whippet, was born after a surf trip to Indonesia. 'I was probably 10 kilos underweight. Then we did a trip to Indonesia, and I was that skinny the nickname stuck. There's a lot worse nicknames than that out there.'

By his late teens, Ryan was surfing well enough to seriously consider a possible professional future. 'To be pushed by the best surfers is a massive bonus,' Ryan says. He looked up to Bronte's finest: world top-10 ranked Tom Whitaker, Luke Hitchings, and Kerrbox. He did the Australian pro junior series and began to tackle the qualifying tour for the big pro surfing leagues, travelling to England and France, but—typical of a young surfer on his first pro-tour adventure—had too much of a good time to give it a proper go. Early the next year, Ryan landed badly while skiing in America with his dad and Cameron, and snapped the anterior cruciate ligament in his left knee. He flew home, had a reconstruction on the knee, and any thoughts of pro surfing went out the window.

While recovering, he spent a surf-free ten months on the Gold Coast doing a diploma in sports management. 'It was kind of weird being away from home and having to look after yourself all that time on crutches. But I loved every minute of it.'

By the time his *Home and Away* role finished, eight years ago, he was over the TV-star thing. 'I was sick of being harassed, going out at night and getting picked on by people. Now, being older makes it easier to deal with.' He has since acted in the Olsen twins movie and had a small part in the award-winning local film *Black Balloon*. But his real efforts have been focused on the job of lifeguard. He's known Aaron Graham, Kerrbox and Harries since childhood. 'I sat down with Box and he said, "Give it a go, if you get on you get on." Five years later I'm still here and loving it.'

He is seasonal, which means full-time nine months of the year, with three months to wind down. 'It is tiring, it's physically taxing so I really appreciate a couple of months off. I go with my old man and do some building, or go overseas for a couple of months ... while I'm still young enough to do that.'

Ryan's first week on the job gave him a thrillseeker's christening: several 30-degree days and an average of 20 rescues a day. He thinks it's easy to take for granted what they do. 'I mean if you're up in the tower and there's a couple of rips raging, and there's five people getting dragged out of one and four getting dragged out of another, and you're there calling the shots, and there's 30 000 people down here and 20 per cent can't swim, and their lives are in your hands, it's a bit daunting sometimes ... And days when it's 8 or 10 feet and there's a few guys out there surfing, and if something goes wrong and I don't go get 'em, nobody else is gonna go get 'em. But it's good fun, the busy days, and when it's big, they're the best. That's what I do it for really. The heavy situations are what you remember, they're the more rewarding ones for me, bringing someone back to life is what it's all about I reckon.'

He's been involved in three such efforts so far. The first was a 25-year-old Japanese guy with an undetected heart problem, who just fell over in a foot of water. Hoppo and Cory Adams, another senior lifeguard, were there, and Ryan was very grateful for their presence. 'I was kinda shitting myself and the more experienced guys took over. I was just doing the small things, radio calls, getting equipment ready, that sort of thing. But it was awesome to watch. Having experienced guys there for your first one is a big moment.'

After *Bondi Rescue Bali*, Ryan stayed on and went surfing for a while; the day after he got home, he went for a pre-work early morning swim at Bronte, and the lifeguards were dragging a body out of the water. 'Fuck! Straight in. He'd committed suicide. We worked on him for 25 minutes ... and ended up getting him back. He died a week or so later in hospital but we felt like we'd done our job, given him every chance he had.'

The drills they do put the processes so firmly in place they're almost automatic. 'You do it all and it's like you don't even know you're doing it. You look up a couple of minutes in and realise everything's done right. That's the level we want everyone to be at down here.'

Ryan thinks Bondi is the 'craziest place I've ever been'. He says, 'Every day's different and on busy days, by 7 p.m. you feel like you're about 100 years old. You're just fried.' He'll tend to go home, then go out for a short surf at Bronte to settle the frazzled nerves. The mental stress of the job is what wears him down, along with exposure from sun and wind. 'Even your sunnies, you can't even see out of the lenses, they're that salty.'

What's the weirdest thing he's seen? 'A guy full-on wanking on the beach. He was doing laps with a camera, taking photos of chicks or whatever, then he went and sat in a chair that he'd rented and fully pulled himself. We caught him, I rang the coppers and they came down, then they said "Come with us", so I did ... and it was so

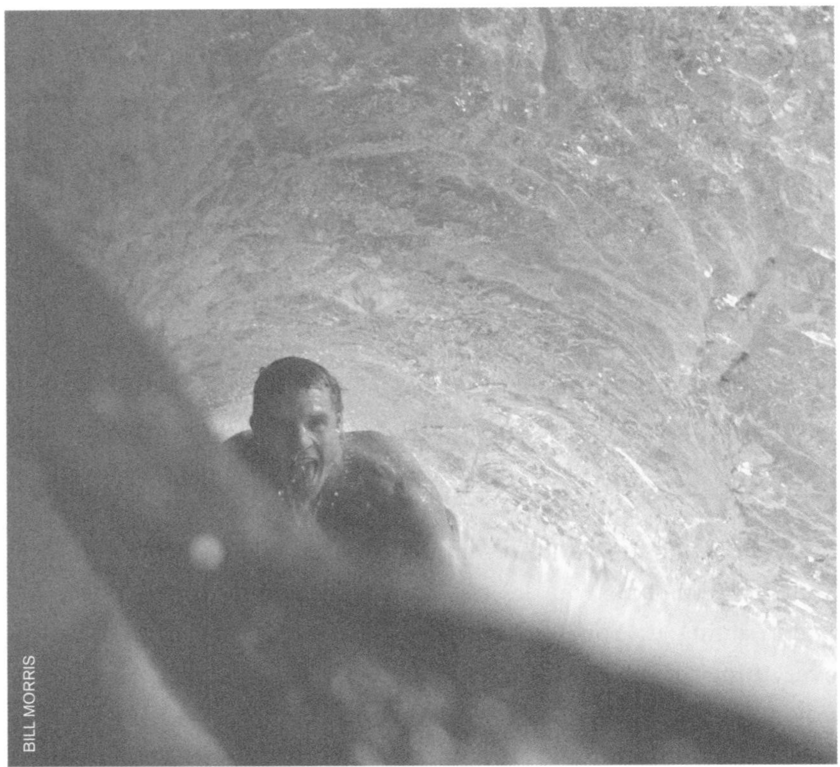
BILL MORRIS

ABOVE Worth smiling about. Whippet snares a rare midday Bondi barrel.

weird, I was almost laughing at the guy, like "What makes you think this is alright doing this, there's kids and mums everywhere and you're having a pull under your towel!"'

Ryan, the clean-cut surfer, is flabbergasted. 'How anyone could think that was possibly acceptable is out of this world.'

The rule is to be as accommodating to the public as you can, as diplomatic as possible, but stand your ground if something's offensive. 'You get out to rescue people and some people are so thankful. They'll hug you and kiss you. But other people you'll get out and rescue them, and it's your fault that they got into trouble in the first place, and it's your fault there's a hundred people on the beach watching them get rescued and dragged in. Some people don't say thanks cos they're embarrassed which is OK, but to have someone say "You let me get into trouble", there's not much you can say. Maybe something like, "Well next time I might not be here to save you ... but have a nice day anyway!"'

Like most of the lifeguards, Ryan thinks the *Bondi Rescue* series has been good for the service, but he points out one downside: crowds. He says they'll get way bigger crowds gathering around any incident, especially if it's serious. 'It's harder to deal with when you've got people yelling "Save him! Fix him up", and it's a spinal or something.'

There are limits to his appetite for thrills. Ryan has yet to participate in a rescue of someone who's gone off the cliff. It's not something he's looking forward to, and for the first time in the conversation, he sounds truly subdued. 'There's been some pretty horrific stories of what the boys have found out there ... when someone's gone off a 100-foot cliff onto rock, they're not gonna be looking that good. I'm sure it'll happen some day. Hopefully not, but ... just try not to look as much as possible. You gotta try and put it out of your head that it's that bad.'

wild stories FROM THE SERVICE

The Ravesi's thief

YOU'VE HEARD OF Ravesi's, right? One of Bondi's nouveau boutique hotel-restaurant combos: $400 a night for a front room, $35 main courses ... and at least once, attempted hideout. Plenty of beach thieves at Bondi. It's an ever-present issue for the lifeguards. They miss a lot, catch a few, mostly turn the task over to the police, who are always on call. One late afternoon Whippet gets a complaint from someone who's been relieved of her possessions; eventually he spots what looks like the thief on the hill to the south. 'I think, "Right, I can catch this guy",' he recalls, and sets off. It turns into a full-on foot race. Trying to evade pursuit, the thief runs straight into Ravesi's and down some internal stairs toward a storeroom, clearly hoping for a backdoor exit. But there's no backdoor. The thief and Whippet end up in this Mexican standoff, fists up and ready to go, till Whippet persuades him that discretion may be the better part of valour: 'I said, "Look we can fight if ya want, but there's four more guys behind me, you've got no chance of getting out of here before the cops come."' The Ravesi's thief is collared.

Paris is burning

WORD GETS OUT that Paris Hilton is in town for various Bondi-related reasons. Whippet is extremely enthusiastic about this highly blonde celeb being in town. 'If she turns up down here I'll be all over her,' he swears to the crew. So it's a super-crowded hot summer's day, Hoppo way up the north end in a rhino, Kerrbox halfway up the beach, Whippet among others in the tower, when Hoppo feels a tap on his arm. It's Paris. 'How are you? Having a nice day?' she asks, and steps past him onto the sand. Hoppo relays the news via radio to the others, and Box reckons he's only just managed to turn his ATV around to point north, when Whippet springs from the tower and is racing through the crowd. Box says, 'Everyone's looking at him thinking, "Jeez, what's gone wrong here? Something big must be happening if a lifeguard's running like that!"' Whippet gets to the sudden throng of people and photographers who've gathered around Ms Hilton, bursts through the pack, and demands, 'Someone get a photo!' Paris ends up parading the beach with a crowd fifteen-deep encircling her famous personage, the lifeguards just shaking their heads.

TOP 8 Things to know for a fun day at Bondi

There's ways to make your beach day fun and easy –just ask the lifeguards.

1. Swim between the flags

It seems basic sort of stuff, but this is number one on every lifeguard's list. 'Bondi's never closed,' says Corey. 'There's always a set of flags somewhere on the beach, so swim there–and follow the signs we put up, they're there to help.

2. Watch your stuff

Don't leave valuables on the sand. Thieves—way more than sharks or rips—are Bondi's biggest torment. 'We catch 'em when we can,' says Hoppo, 'but it's a big beach with a lot of ways to escape.'

3. Sunscreen!

It's amazing how many people forget it, or even worse, don't think of it at all ... till it's too late. The boys still recall the person from Birmingham, England, who thought he was dying of some waterborne disease because 'I'm red all over, and it stings!'

4. Don't drink alcohol

For one thing, it's illegal to have alcoholic drink containers on the beach at Bondi. For another, drinking leads to anti-social behaviour, which in a crowd of 50,000, doesn't work very well. For a third, drinking alcohol causes dehydration, which leads us to the next point ...

5. Drink plenty of water

'It's amazing how much fluid the body loses on a sunny day on the beach,' says Harries. 'You can't afford to dehydrate on a hot day.'

6. Treat other beach-goers with respect

This one's obvious. At Bondi, as in most places, you'll get what you give in this department. 'There's space for everyone,' says Hoppo.

7. Approach the lifeguards—and be aware of where to find them if you need help

'We're the shepherds of the beach,' says Tom. 'We're totally OK about you coming up and talking to us. Get a photo with a lifeguard! It'll be fine.'

8. Relax and enjoy it!

'And bring a friend,' advises Reidy. 'It's always better fun to swim with someone else.'

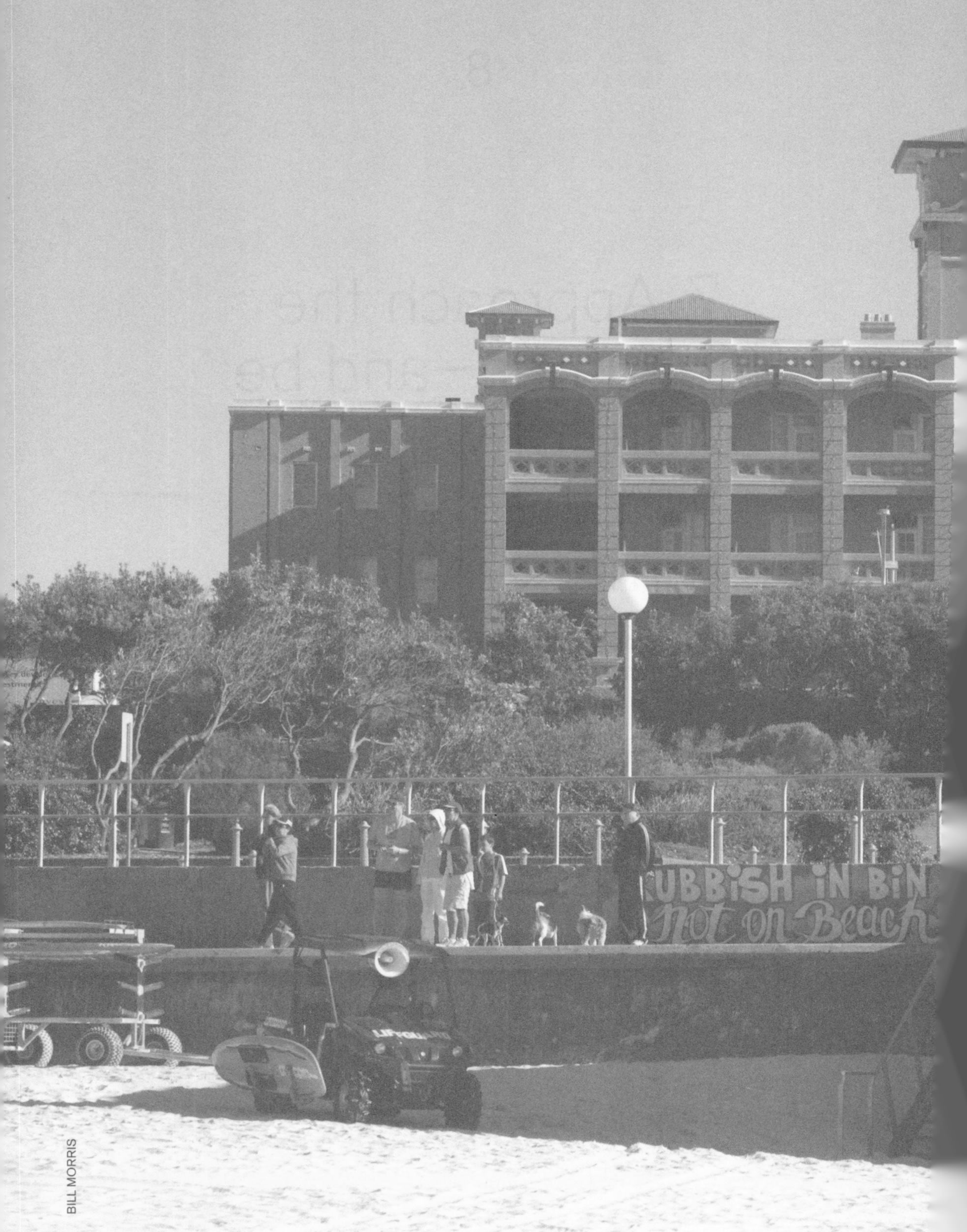

BILL MORRIS

8
EVENTS OF A SEASON

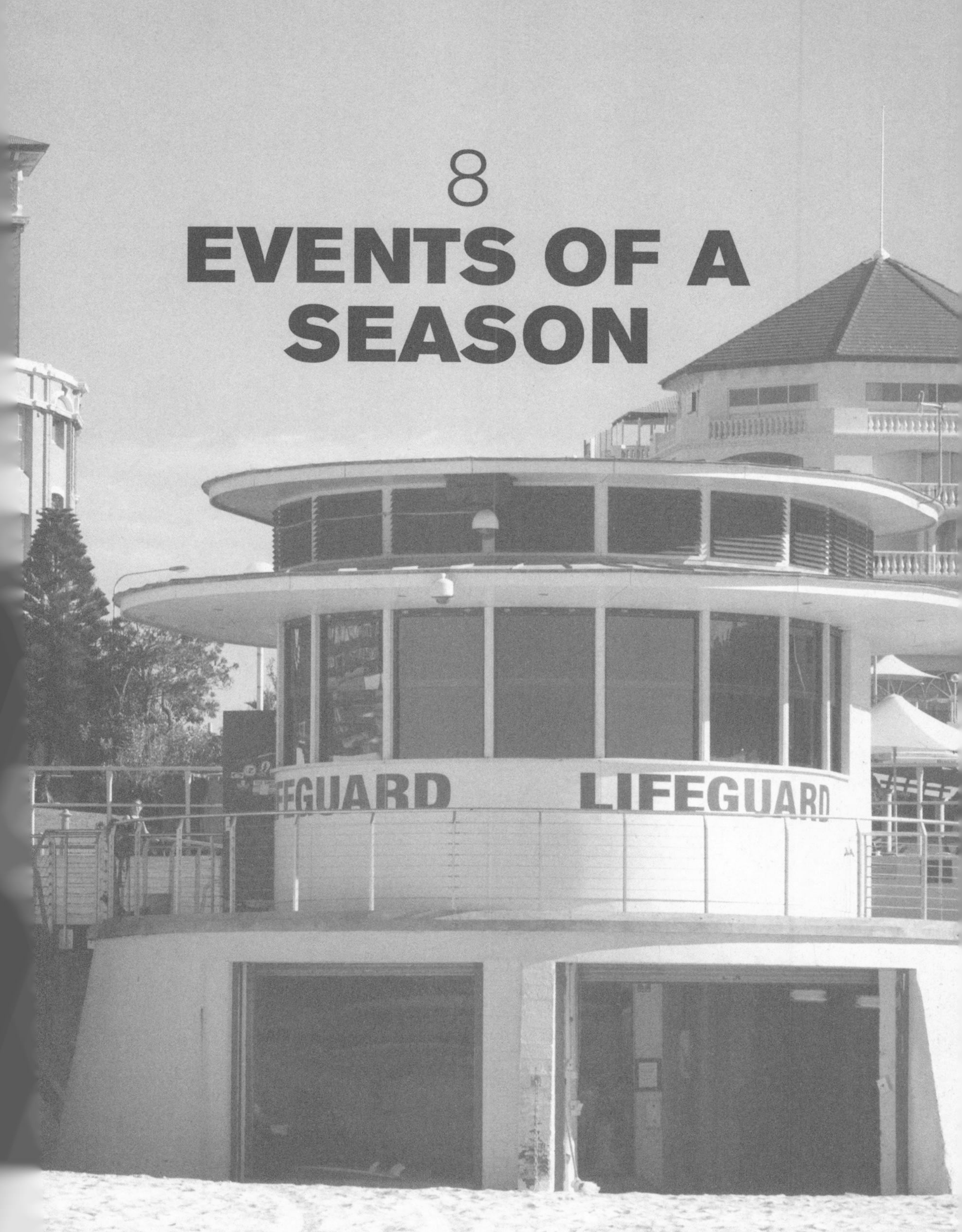

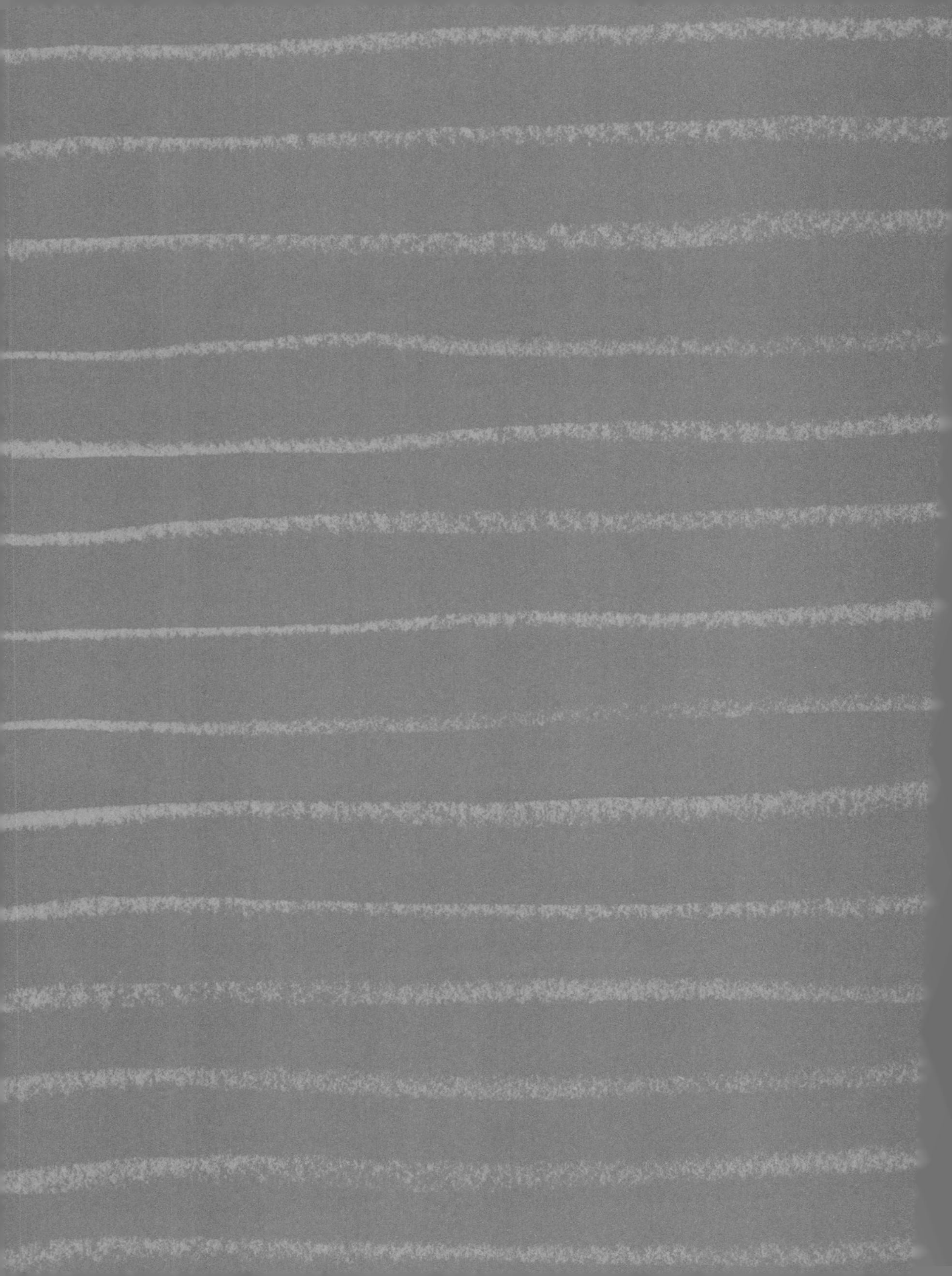

Highlights and lowlights of Bondi 2009

Spring, summer, autumn ... a nine-month arc during which each year, the Aussie east coast buds, blooms, shines, and gently declines. Even if you're not a die-hard beach lover, chances are you'll find yourself wandering along a stretch of sand somewhere during these months, having tossed away the trappings of politer society for that salty cool hedonism Australians have pretty much patented. For most of us, it's a magic time—what other nation just sorta stops functioning for the month after Christmas, simply by mutual consent? For the Bondi lifeguard crew, it's a different tale every year; along with the fun, they get to deal with the wild stuff, the bleak, the frightening and the dramatic, the stuff most of us never have to see. Here's a look at the bigger moments of 2009.

Suicide at Bronte

22 September 2008: It's the spring equinox along the Australian east coast, and fittingly for the date, an extraordinarily clear morning unveils itself across Bronte Bay. One of those days most of us feel lucky to be alive, which makes what happens even more painfully ironic. Without a sound or scream, unseen at first by anyone, a man jumps from the cliff top at the southern end of the bay. His body misses the rock shelf below and hits the ocean surface with what one witness later describes as a 'heavy thudding plop'.

Some time later, perhaps 30 seconds, he appears to regain consciousness and signals weakly for help, then slumps back underwater. People up on the cliff are dialling 000 and watching in horror. On the beach, Corey Oliver is on duty and sees Harries bolting towards the tower. The pair grab boards and start motoring. 'We paddled our guts out to try and get there and as we got there we were "Oh my God",' recalls Corey. 'He hadn't hit the rocks so there wasn't anything obviously wrong with him, but his neck was all swollen, just instant trauma. We put him across two boards and tried to paddle him in as far as we could, then the boys put him on the ski and got him in. There was myself, Harries and Maxy the trainee … I felt sorry for Maxy to have to see something so intense.' By some trick of fortune or coincidence, or maybe just because the waves are pretty good, a number of guards are at the beach, including Whippet; they respond swiftly and within a couple of minutes there are eleven of them working on the suicide. Somehow, radically against the odds, they manage to claw him back into the world of heartbeats. They don't know his story, the history of depression; they don't know then that he'll eventually die in hospital as a result of his injuries. 'I think the ambos were really surprised we kept him alive,' says Corey. 'I think he was on life support for four or five days. The parents were ringing Harries quite a bit and I think it was doing his head in a bit, but he was really good with them. For the boys, professionally, to know something so traumatic had happened and yet we'd kept him alive, was a real boost.'

The No-Doz kid

A cool afternoon, four days after the Bronte suicide. Whippet is at radio central up in the Bondi tower. A new boy, Luke Daniels, is cruising south along the sand on one of the rhinos. Kerrbox, Kris Yates and a few other guards are around, off-duty and on. Luke radios in the first concern of his lifeguarding career: 'There's a man with a dog down here, what should we do about him?'

Don't be too concerned, advises Whippet, with a suppressed chuckle, thinking to himself that the rookie is very eager. Then the radio crackles again: 'Unconscious patient.' Whippet does a double-take—'What?' he queries Luke. 'I've got an unconscious patient!' comes the confirmation. Luke has seen a head attached to an unresponsive body, floating in a rip not far from the central flagged area, and dives in after it. The lifeguards have a signal—if something's going down, someone will flip the shark alarm a couple of times just quickly, and if anyone's around they know to come running.

Whippet flips the alarm, grabs a defibrillator and takes off towards the scene. Luke has done superbly; he's already with the patient, supporting the body while Kerrbox and several other guards are sprint-swimming towards them. The victim turns out to be a seventeen-year-old boy on the brink of his Higher School Certificate exams; he'd been taking No-Doz pills to excess in order to stay up with his studies, and tension and the lack of sleep caught up with him. He'd had a seizure. 'I got there and Luke was doing mouth-to-mouth on him, thumping his chest, he had foam coming out and all sorts,' says Whippet (drowning victims who've inhaled water sometimes 'foam at the mouth' as the detergent-like lung lining fizzes out). 'I told Luke, "Mate, stop breathing into him, I'll get a mask on him", and Luke had this look on his face, like, "Fuck! What the fuck's going on?!" Luckily Kerrbox was swimming just 50 metres down. Within a minute or two we had seven lifeguards working on him and we got him back in about a minute. But if it wasn't for Luke's quick actions he coulda been in a lot worse way.'

Two dramatic events within a few days of each other … it feels as if the tone has been set for a big season. Yet oddly enough, the next few months produce little but small surf, warm days and few rescues. The main issue for the year will be crowds.

Save us!

A baking day in the hottest Sydney January on record. Ten thousand people are on the beach, 20,000, 30,000, more. The surf conditions are relatively safe, but with such a huge crowd, even a small incident metastasises into something weird, distracting, almost uncontrollable; when someone hits the bottom and has to be brought to the beach for treatment for a suspected spinal injury, the lifeguards are surrounded by clusters of unruly humanity, jostling and yelling, 'Save him! Fix him up!'

Outside the break, Kerrbox is on jet-ski duty, following hard-to-hear radio instructions from the tower, when he spots three swimmers who seem to be in trouble. Their hands are up and they're asking for assistance. Box pulls up to the three and gets them onto the ski's rescue sled and begins driving back to shore; when he takes a quick look to check on his passengers, they're standing up on the sled, waving to the TV cameras. 'I dropped them off near the beach and said to 'em, "Please don't signal unless you need help, it's too crowded for that today".'

Twenty minutes later he sees the same three swimmers, hands up, waving for help; races across, loads them onto the sled, and exactly the same thing happens. It's just a big joke. Box bites his tongue, drops them off, and leaves them with another request to lay off. Sure enough another 20 minutes down the track, there they are again, surrounded by other swimmers and waving, seemingly desperate for help. 'I wanted to tell 'em to piss off ... but the public who's watching it all happen don't know these idiots are just playing up. You can't really walk away, you've still gotta rescue 'em, but at the same time, they're distracting us from what we're supposed to be doing.' Box radios the beach this time to let the crew know there are some tricksters around the place.

Later in the day, the same people engage in more offensive behaviour towards other beach-goers, and cause lifeguards to call the police. Kerrbox worries that he's seeing a pattern emerge—that Bondi's modern crowds are so fragmented, chaos now is almost inevitable. 'If there's an incident now, people flock to it, they get in the way. It's one drawback of us being well-known; they've seen us on TV and they know we're gonna rescue 'em no matter what.'

Box's rock ride

It starts off very easily—a classic late January day, with a small pulse of surf running across the beach slightly north-to-south, feeding the rip next to Icebergs. The day is no threat to anyone who stays up in the centre flagged area, but it turns foul for three girls who jump in at the south end and are sucked quickly out past the rocks. The old firm of Kerrbox and Hoppo are on the case; Box is first there and finds himself locked into a sort of washing-machine cycle.

The small swell is focusing in on the rocks, and the rip is pulling across behind them, which locks them into a hole of deep water in a reef crevice off the south headland. 'I had the three girls,' recalls Box, 'and we were being pushed into the back of Icebergs. I palmed one of 'em off on Hoppo and we started trying to work our way back out of the hole. But we didn't get a break. There was set after set coming down on us, and we just couldn't make any ground.

Box's head is suddenly full of nightmare scenarios: what if his patient slides off? She'll be shredded on the barnacles!

'Young Bacon came out on the ski but he couldn't reach us.' Kerrbox, the lifelong surfer, makes the kind of decision that runs against his every instinct; he turns his board—and his patient—back towards the rocks. 'I had no option,' he reckons. 'I just yelled, "Hang the fuck on!" In a way it was probably the most dangerous thing I've ever done. But I really had no option.'

Box slides back on the board, trying frantically to keep its nose up as they're picked up by a piece of whitewater and hurled towards the rock platform. His head's suddenly full of the nightmare scenarios: What if the girl slides off as they hit? She'll be shredded on the barnacles! Instead, they're overtaken by the most ridiculous piece of luck. The board touches down on a soft blanket of cunjevoi and eelgrass, and Box and his unsuspecting patient walk away to safety. Not even the board sustains any damage. Box can't believe it. 'It was funny, because before the rescue, Hoppo and I were sitting up the north end of the beach and talking about how we hadn't done a rescue behind the rocks for ages. We'd talked our way through exactly the same scenario ... then it actually happened! Not quite the way we'd talked about it though.'

The shark attack

The season's quiet ends—along with the crowds—at around 8 p.m. on 12 February. A 33-year-old surfer named Glenn Orgias is out at the south end, along with 20 or so others, in a rising choppy easterly swell. The water is discoloured thanks to the first rain in seven weeks. A shark, later identified via injury analysis as a small great white, snatches at Glenn's left hand and nearly tears it clean off at the wrist. It's the defining event of the entire Sydney summer, yet the lifeguards have been off the beach for half an hour; they begin to find out via news broadcasts and text messages. Reidy sees Box's number pop up on his phone a few times, but is determined to ignore it, thinking it must be a call to Thursday-night carnage of some kind. Eventually he opens a text and sees the words 'Shark attack at Bondi!! Can't believe it.'

Neither can anyone else. Ryan Clark is on a snowboarding trip to Japan. His girlfriend sends him an email that says, 'You're never surfing Bondi again!' Whippet's seen a shark at Bondi once himself, out past Ben Buckler, but he's always had the thought tucked away where most good surfers keep it: 'I'm pretty sweet with the shark thing. I know they're there but you're more likely to get hit by a car.'

The sentiment isn't shared by most of the rest of Sydney; the city's media responds as if an act of terrorism has occurred. Hoppo wears much of the aftermath of the shark incident, spending more or less the entire next day doing media interviews. People had been bumped a few times in the days beforehand, and there was at least one further positive sighting on Sunday.

Hoppo figures that the drama will probably pass after the weather dies down. Numbers on the beach have been low, but the weather's been bad in any case. He says, 'It'll be funny to see what happens when things clear up—dunno if anyone'll be swimming the bay.' He's right in a way: The beach doesn't change much, but out in the water, the vibe is very strange. The hardcore local surfers whom the lifeguards depend on for accurate info and feedback are on edge and jumpy; one later reports seeing a shark take a seabird off the surface just outside the south end sandbar a few days after the attack. The media doesn't help matters; one newspaper crew shoots a photo of a shark working a school of mullet 20 metres away from a bodyboard, and runs the pic on the front page next day—without telling the lifeguards. That move 'jumps the shark' with the lifeguards; suddenly they are seeing the ugly side of media. 'We told 'em, "Don't ever try anything like that again",' says a grim Kerrbox.

Despite lengthy surgery, doctors are unable to save Glenn Orgias's hand; it's amputated a month or so later. The news doesn't even make the front page.

Body at Bondi

Early March is often one of the nicest times of the year at Bondi: still warm and clear, yet without the hectic energies of midsummer. The pleasures of early autumn escape Corey Oliver when he, along with fellow lifeguard Troy, are dispatched via jet ski to retrieve a human body that's been spotted floating offshore.

When the pair arrive, they find the body in a state of rigor mortis; it's clearly been in the water overnight. Again, they have no idea what's happened. The water police have asked that the body be kept offshore until they arrive, so for more than half an hour they remain 800 metres off the beach, with the body, Troy keeping it secured on the sled with his own body weight. They sit and talk for a while together until the police boat shows up to relieve them. To Corey, it's an act of respect for the victim—to deliberately avoid exposing it to merely curious eyes. 'For me, I've seen this stuff before,' he says, recalling both the early season suicide and an event from the year before, when a girl had jumped to her death at Bronte. 'A lot of people might think I'm a bit weird, driving out that far, but I take a bit of pride in that situation; it's sensitive and dealing with it in the right manner is important.'

The rock fishermen deaths

Late in the season, autumn's bell is swung. The first great surf of the season is forecast to arrive in the afternoon of Friday 24 April. It does, in large sets of waves with long lulls—lulls long enough to tempt a rock fisherman into the wrong place on Ben Buckler. He's reported missing, but a late search reveals nothing. Deano, who is rostered lead guy on Saturday morning, gets a referral to assist in the morning's continued search. By now the swell has risen further to a solid 2 to 3 metres, sweeping from the east off Ben Buckler down towards Bronte. At 8.25 a.m., the water police call to say they've found the body. Two lifeguards, Beardy and Michael 'Mouse' Jansen, pull their ski up next to the police boat, and notice something astounding: traces of foam are flowing from the fisherman's mouth. How could it be, if the guy has been dead in the water all night? In fact, it is a different fisherman altogether—this one having been swept off the rocks only a few minutes previously.

The lifeguards realise he may be recoverable. Mouse leaps off his ski and onto the police boat to attempt a resuscitation, but without effective equipment—the boat has no oxygen and its defibrillator doesn't seem to be functioning—he's going backwards. He and Beardy desperately urge the police to head for the beach, where the crew can jump to it with oxygen and defib, while another lifeguard ski races out with more equipment. But instead, the police choose to evacuate the victim using the Westpac helicopter—which ironically is down a paramedic staff thanks to budget cuts. The tangle of decision-making adds up the wrong way. In the ten minutes it takes to transfer him from the boat to an ambulance at Watson's Bay via helicopter, the fisherman dies. The lifeguards are furious and frustrated. 'The bottom line is that he shouldn't have died,' says Deano soberly. The original subject of the search remains missing.

The local makes it back

Sunday 26 April. Funny how things happen in clusters. Deano is on duty again, writing reports from yesterday's fisherman disaster, while several of the others are on jet skis overseeing a 5-kilometre ocean swim race from Coogee to Bondi. The surf's much smaller and the local longboard club is having their monthly contest. By late morning there are eight lifeguards in the tower, hanging out: Deano, Hoppo, Whippet, Reidy and several others.

Suddenly there's a commotion: a couple of beginners are struggling with somebody not far offshore, and a surf lifesaver is running towards the scene. Dean and Whippet are on one of the rhinos and on the scene in 30 seconds. The victim turns out to be 61-year-old Tim Pearson, a long-time local resident whom all the boys have known for ages. He's been surfing in the contest and suffered a heart attack. Deano organises moving the patient up to dry sand, and swiftly the defibrillator and oxygen are deployed. Reidy counts the cycles, pumping Tim's chest while Whippet puts oxygen into him. They run through four compression/breath cycles, about two minutes' effort, when the defib announces in its robotic voice, 'Administer shock—stand clear'. Boom—the volts are delivered. The boys dive in to keep the cycles up, then suddenly Tim is alive, gasping for air. They keep the oxygen bag on him as the ambulance crew arrives. 'He was hypoxic [suffering from lack of oxygen in body tissues] so he was being quite aggressive, trying to get up,' recounts Reidy. 'His mates were in his face telling him, "Calm down mate, you're with the lifeguards, everything's OK". The last thing he said as they carted him away was "Make sure somebody gets my board!" We thought that was a good sign.'

The boys dive in, then suddenly Tim is alive, gasping for air. 'Make sure somebody gets my board!' he says.

Sure enough, Tim spends a day in intensive care, then he's sitting up and doing well. 'They all matter,' says Reidy. 'But when it's someone you see every day and say hello to, it makes a difference.'

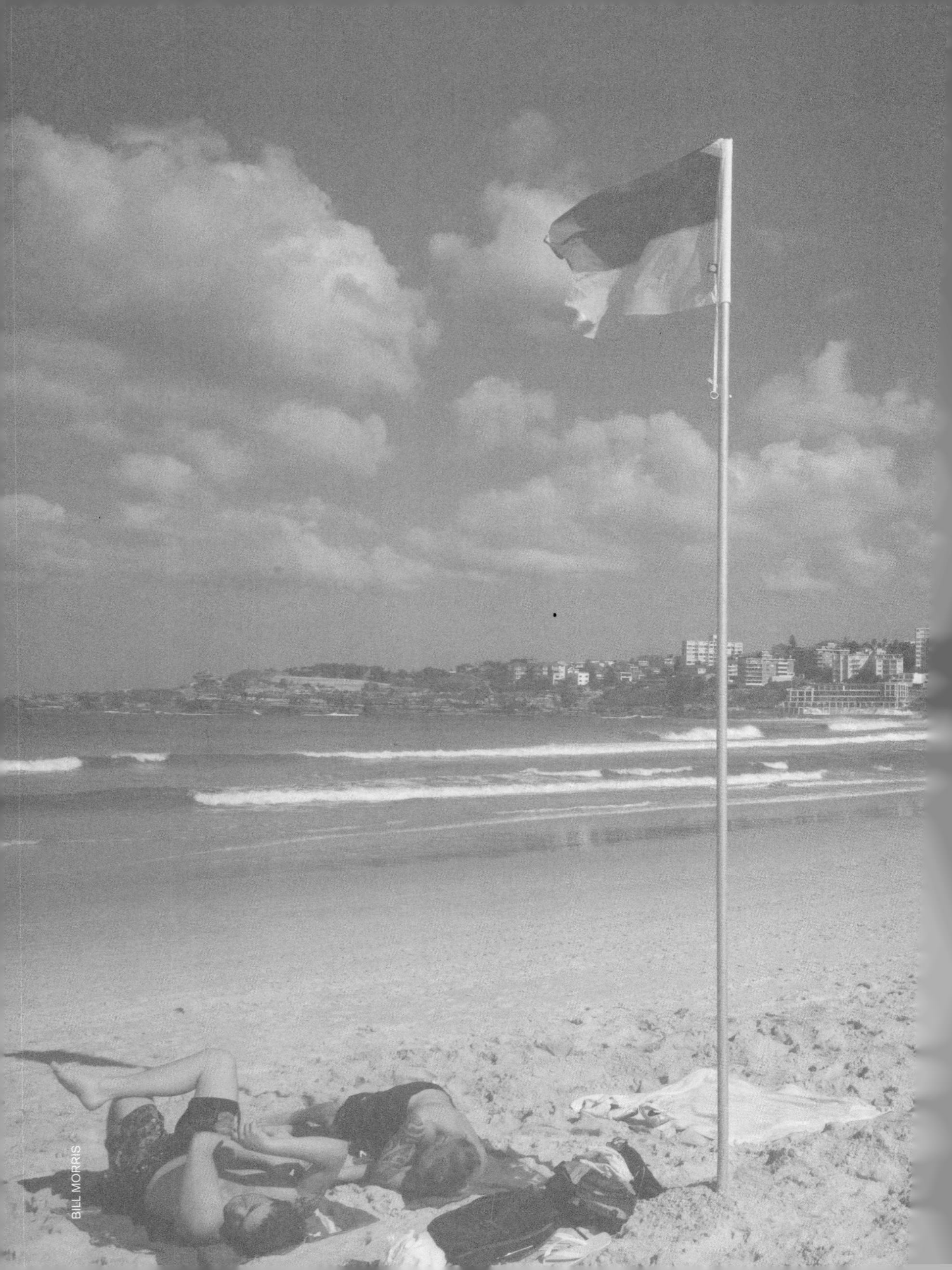

BILL MORRIS

9
SOME FINAL TIPS FROM THE BOYS

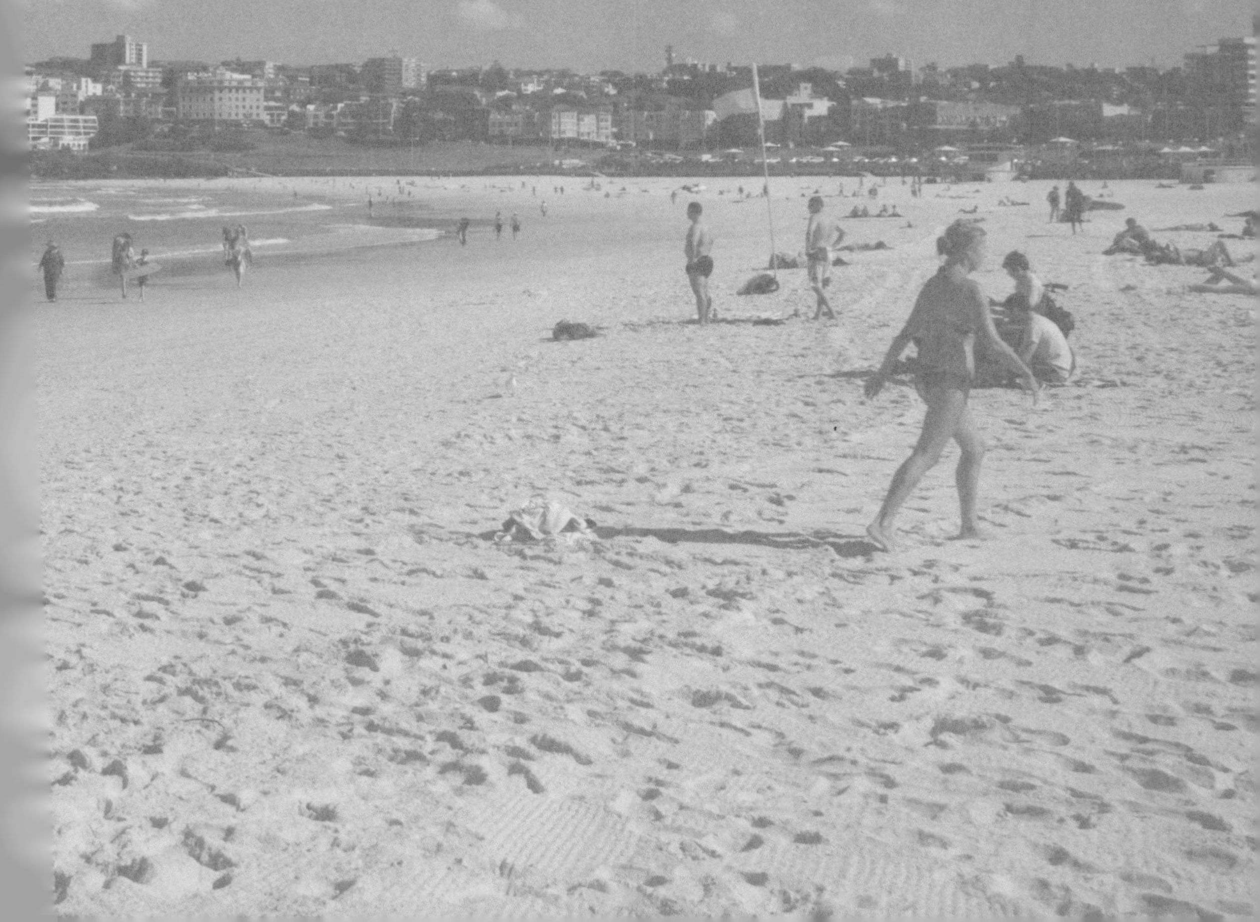

What the guards don't know ain't worth knowing

Like lifeguards everywhere, the Bondi crew live in the hope that you'll never have to call on them for help. They're constantly acting on the belief that prevention is better than cure. With that in mind, they've provided you with the following tips and tricks to help you stay out of trouble at the beach—and what to do if trouble just happens to find you ...

Check you have sunscreen and sun protection

Sunburn is always better prevented than suffered. If you do get yourself burned, it'll show up as a persistent reddening of the exposed skin and it'll be tender to the touch. If you get badly sunburned, even moving the sunburned body part will sting.

If you do get sunburned, stay out of the sun, drink plenty of water (if you've been sunburned, you'll also be dehydrated), have a cold shower, wear light clothing, and apply an aloe vera-based moisturiser. The sunburn's effects will recede over a couple of days and may result in peeling of the burned skin's surface layer; keep the new skin protected from sunlight until the peeling has disappeared.

Watch out for bluebottles

Bluebottles are tiny marine colonies made up of bubble-like floats, digestive organs, and long single tentacles covered in small, wicked stinging cells. If your exposed skin comes into contact with those cells, they'll release a microscopic barb and inject you with a very irritating and painful mix of chemicals.

'Bluey' stings can be treated immediately with ice or a simple anti-irritant remedy like Stingose. The stinging sensation usually passes within a half-hour, but itching can go on for a while. To prevent this, get home and have a warm shower for around ten minutes—the hot water breaks down the bluebottle's complex stinging substance.

In rare cases, people suffer anaphylactic shock reaction to bluey stings; the reaction can be life-threatening, so keep an eye on any first-time victim.

some final tips from the boys

Pay attention to the beach signage

It'll save you time, energy, and maybe the need to be rescued if you pay attention to signs and flags on the beach. When it comes to this, you're your own best lifeguard.

Avoid beach thieves!

Don't take valuables down to the sands with you; lock them in your car or leave them at home. Don't rely on friends to keep an eye on your gear—why make them responsible? Don't give thieves an even break.

Approach a lifeguard if you need help

Always feel free to approach lifeguards with any issues or problems that might arise during your visit to the beach. If they can't directly help, they'll point you to the people who can.

Join Nippers

All the *Bondi Rescue* lifeguards know: Surf lifesaving's junior activities are the perfect way for any kid to gain the water skills that'll make their surf and beach lives a dream.

Nippers programs are run by individual surf lifesaving clubs between October and March at most Australian urban beaches and many regional locations. To check for your local surf club's Nipper program go to the official SLSA website, www.slsa.asn.au, and click on Resources, then Nippers. Or just go straight to your nearest surf club and ask any member!

www.bondirescue.com

www.bondirescuelifeguards.com

How to perform CPR

Here's a guide to a critical lifeguard skill that could one day save someone's life—whether it's your best mate's or a complete stranger's. CPR—cardio-pulmonary resuscitation—is a technique that keeps the heart and lungs working when a person's body can't do the job itself. To do it well, you'll need to find out just how it works.

Every cell in your body needs a regular supply of oxygen to keep functioning. Your body also needs to flush away by-products of oxygen use. This work is done by the lungs, which absorb oxygen into the blood and expel carbon dioxide, and the heart, which pumps oxygen-rich blood from the lungs around the body and draws 'used' blood back to the lungs for resupply.

CPR combines external breathing with chest compressions designed to put oxygen in the blood and move it around the body. It can keep key organs—most importantly the brain—ticking over until the body is able to restart the job itself.

Lifeguards and other professionals use high-end stuff like a defibrillator and an Oxy-Viva pure oxygen delivery system to do the job. But they still have to learn old-fashioned hands-on CPR and, let's face it, you're unlikely to own either a defibrillator or an Oxy-Viva delivery system. So let's walk through the plain old manual method. This is a simplified sequence of events. It's coded in a simple acronym—DR ABCDE.

D is for Danger—to others and to yourself. Check the scene for possible risks such as exposed electrical wires or broken glass. Aside from further danger to your patient, it's really important to make sure you're not placing yourself in danger; if you're also hurt or somehow rendered useless, then what chance has your patient got? Call 000 immediately.

R is for Response—Check to see if the patient is responding. Talk to them; if you get no response, gently grasp the hands or shoulders of your patient and squeeze. If the patient responds, he or she will be conscious, and there'll be no need for CPR.

A is for Airway—Check if the patient's airway is blocked by anything. An unconscious patient may have a lapsed tongue falling back into his or her throat; if the patient is just out of the water, there might be seaweed in there, vomit, anything. Kneel beside your patient and tilt the head slightly back—this straightens the airway line from mouth to lungs—and lift open the mouth, using a one-hand grip on your patient's jaw and chin, to check.

B is for Breathing—Look, listen and feel for evidence of the patient breathing. Look at the possible rise and fall of the chest; listen for any sounds from the patient's mouth and nose; feel the chest and ribcage for any movement. If the patient is breathing, place in the recovery position—patient on side, head facing downhill if possible and supported by lower shoulder/arm, other arm loosely crooked across the lower arm, and upper leg loosely crooked over the lower leg to support—and watch closely until help arrives. If not, then clear the airway and commence rescue breathing.

Rescue breathing involves you using your own breath to inflate your patient's lungs. It works because you only use about a quarter of the oxygen in any given breath, so there's plenty left for your patient's bloodstream to scavenge. To breathe, keep the patient's head tilted, with one of your hands on the forehead and finger and thumb pinching the nose, the other hand pulling the mouth open with that one-hand grip on jaw and chin. Lock your mouth over the patient's and breathe out firmly and evenly; it should take a bit less than a second. Then lift your mouth away and watch the chest for signs of it having risen and fallen, and feel for air escaping out of the patient's mouth.

Give two breaths this way, then ...

C is for Compressions—If the patient is not breathing and there are no signs of life, commence chest compressions.

Compressions involve you using your body weight to push down and 'squeeze' the heart, forcing it to pump and draw blood around the body. Kneeling next to your patient, pick a point in the centre of his or her chest, roughly in line with his or her underarms. You should be able to feel a big bone (it's called the sternum) under your fingers. Now place the heel of one hand on the spot, brace the wrist with your other hand, and lean down to compress, then back up to release. Do this quickly and firmly. The whole movement, down and up, should take less than a second. It should compress your patient's chest about a third of the way through. Make sure you fully withdraw your weight when releasing each compression—it's just as important that the heart refills with blood between each squeeze, in order to keep it flowing.

You should alternate breaths and compressions at a rate of two breaths to 30 compressions, with cycles happening at a rate of two per minute. This is the actual CPR process. It should be continued until your patient shows signs of recovery, or until qualified emergency assistance arrives.

CPR is hard physical work; if two of you are available and know what to do, take turns on the compressions, switching roles every four cycles.

D is for Defibrillation—Since you don't have one ...

some final tips from the boys

E is for Emergency services—Call 000.

If performing CPR on an infant less than a year old, modify compressions to use two fingers and do not use the head tilt. If the patient is a young child, use one hand or two if needed. In both cases, try for the one-third compression of the chest cavity as a guide to how much pressure is needed.

Remember: 2 breaths to 30 compressions.

BILL MORRIS

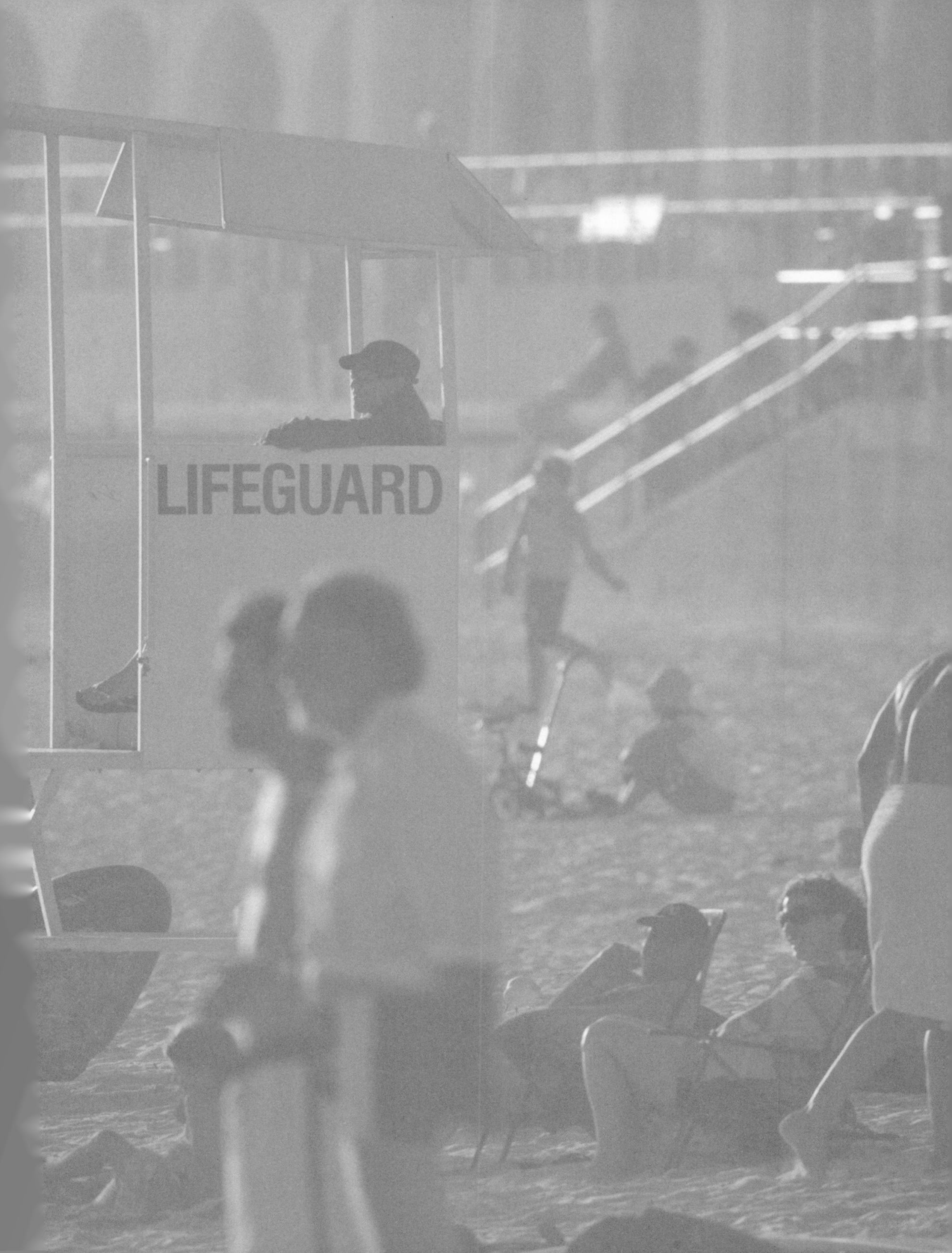
LIFEGUARD

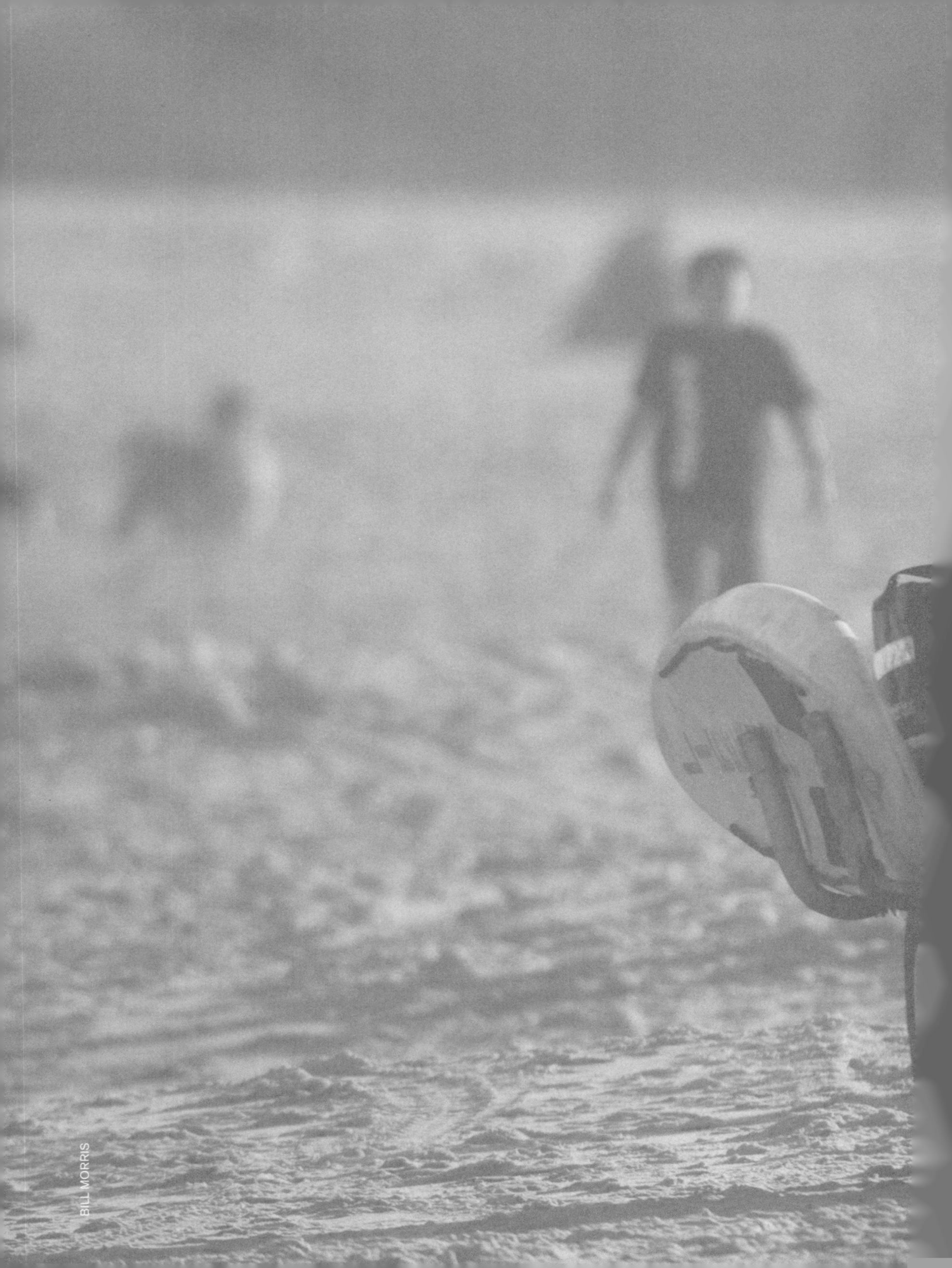

BILL MORRIS

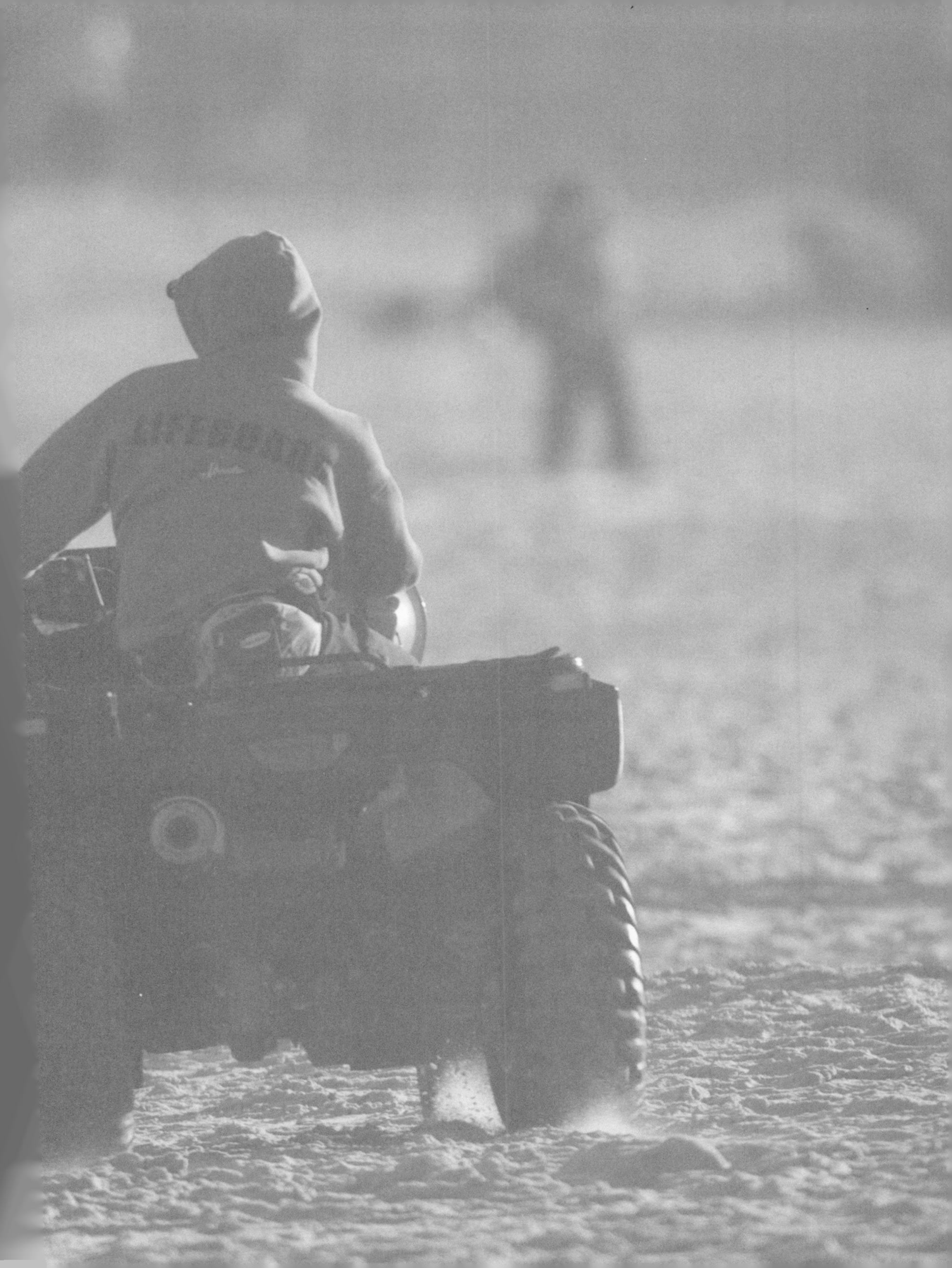

ACKNOWLEDGMENTS

The author would like to thank all the lifeguards, young and young at heart, who assisted him in understanding their role in Bondi's fascinating surf and beach culture. Top of the list go Hoppo, Box, Reidy, Harries, Tom, Whippet, Corey and Deano, but it also includes Harry Nightingale Jr, Terry McDermott, the Graham brothers (Aaron and Kobi), Mouse, Aaron, Brad Malyon, Itchy and all the rest of the Waverley lifeguard crew. Especially we'd like to thank Lawrie Williams for his patience in explaining the Bondi lifeguards' history and for helping us with photos from earlier times.

The book wouldn't be complete without a big thanks to *Bondi Rescue*'s TV production crew, including producer Ben Davies, for their unfailing good nature and helpfulness. Generally speaking, there's a great spirit between the crew and the lifeguards. In the line of duty the crew's had a broken leg, drowned audio mixer, severely torn hamstring, and more than a few rescues spotted while lifeguards have been attending to other duties. We'd also like to acknowledge executive producer Michael Cordell of Cordell Jigsaw. Not only is Michael a great narration writer and storyteller, he's also lived the better part of his life at Bondi, making him heavily invested in the integrity of the program.

Harries would like to thank his long-time girlfriend, Rebecca, who stood by him for many years. Whippet thanks his mum and dad for all the support, and offers a massive thanks to the whole lifeguard service—you're the best bunch of boys he could ever have worked with. Thanks to Bill Morris for his fine images of the crew and their amazing workplace.

Many thanks also to Jude McGee, Louise Thurtell and Elissa Baillie of Allen & Unwin, who saw the book's potential, to Alexandra Nahlous who proofread and guided it, and to Deborah Pearson, who shepherded it all home calmly and with much forbearance.

May you all get a wave at Bondi—without needing a rescue!

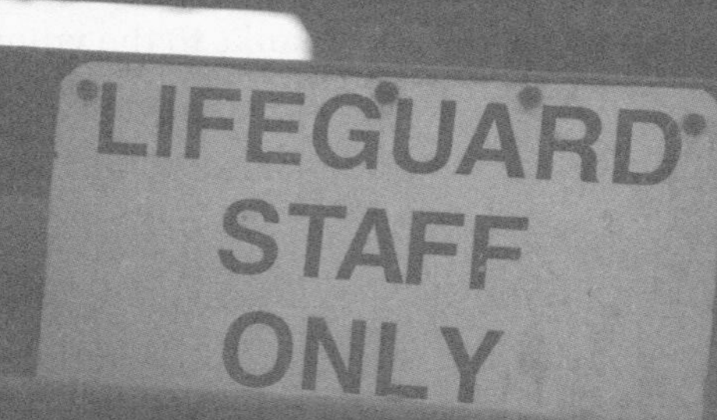
LIFEGUARD
STAFF
ONLY